Women Who Sell Sex

Elizabeth Krumrei Mancuso ·
Bennett E. Postlethwaite

Women Who Sell Sex

A Review of Psychological Research With Clinical Implications

Springer

Elizabeth Krumrei Mancuso
Social Science Division
Pepperdine University
Malibu, CA, USA

Bennett E. Postlethwaite
Business Administration Division
Pepperdine University
Malibu, CA, USA

ISBN 978-3-030-47026-5 ISBN 978-3-030-47027-2 (eBook)
https://doi.org/10.1007/978-3-030-47027-2

This Springer imprint is published by the registered company Springer Nature Switzerland AG
The registered company address is: Gewerbestrasse 11, 6330 Cham, Switzerland

Acknowledgments

We would like to warmly thank our students and research assistants who have worked with us on this topic over the years, including Rosemond Travis, Chelsie Cost, Sarah Zhang, Steven Zhou, and Theresa Brown.

Contents

About the Authors

Elizabeth Krumrei Mancuso is Associate Professor of Psychology at Pepperdine University's Seaver College of Letters, Arts, and Sciences. Her Ph.D. is in clinical psychology and she is licensed as a psychologist in California. She has been primary investigator on a number of grant-funded research projects and has published in the areas of the psychology of religion, virtues, and prostitution. She co-authored the monograph, *Faith from a Positive Psychology Perspective*.

Bennett E. Postlethwaite is Associate Professor of Organizational Behavior and Management at Pepperdine University's Seaver College of Letters, Arts, and Sciences. His research focuses on personality, employee selection, and managing groups and teams. He has a Ph.D. in Organizational Behavior and Human Resource Management from the University of Iowa and an M.Sc. in Health Management from Imperial College London.

Chapter 1
The Psychology of Selling Sex: An Introduction

Although it is difficult to accurately estimate the total size of the commercial sex industry, there is a broad consensus that the industry is large, profitable, and growing (Weitzer, 2010). This book focuses on one slice of commercial sex: private, in-person, consensual sex acts exchanged between a woman and a paying customer. It goes by many names: prostitution, sex work, hooking, whoring, escorting, hustling, and has various legal statuses across the world. Public policy debates about selling sex focus on many concerns, such as public health, community safety, human rights, women's rights, violence, oppression, and human trafficking. Psychological views of selling sex can range broadly, from the idea that selling sex is intrinsically traumatizing and results in mental health problems to the idea that selling sex can be consistent with a positive expression of sexuality. In recent times, popular attention has focused on women marketing themselves on personal websites, offering more in common between the commercial sale of sex and conventional service industries. In an age in which websites and apps are making the sale of sex more accessible to a larger proportion of society, questions about the psychological motivations and mental health correlates of this activity are particularly pertinent. This book explores these themes by reviewing the empirical literature about women who sell sex.

Before delving into the empirical research in subsequent chapters of the book, we cover four preliminary matters in this chapter. First, we present the goals of this book. Next, we offer background information about the methodology and terminology used throughout the book. Then, we review the primary ideological stances toward selling sex and explain how these viewpoints inform the topics covered in this volume. Finally, we highlight a few methodological issues in the primary research of women who sell sex that are important to have in perspective when learning about this literature.

E. Krumrei Mancuso and B. E. Postlethwaite, *Women Who Sell Sex*,
https://doi.org/10.1007/978-3-030-47027-2_1

The Goals of this Book

Topics Covered

This book is not about the act or institution of selling sex. Rather, it is about the psychological experiences of women who sell sex. This book will review the literature on a number of psychological concepts related to selling sex, including motivation, stigma, stress, coping, and mental health. Quite an extensive body of scholarly work exists on this topic. The purpose of this book is to summarize themes from the research in order to offer a brief introduction to the topic with implications for mental health professionals and directions for future research.

The goal is to evaluate these topics among women who have made some level of deliberate choice to sell sex. This raises an important question regarding freedom of choice. Some philosophers, theorists, and researchers have argued that consensual sex can exist only when there is economic and social equality between the persons involved. Under this theory, women who sell sex from a position of low economic or social power are likely to experience coercion, calling into question the voluntary nature of their encounters. Some believe all or the majority of women who sell sex do not have a choice, or they have a choice so constrained that it should not be considered a true choice (e.g., Raymond, 2013). For example, Moran (2012), a woman who describes herself as having been prostituted between the ages of 15–22, wrote in her blog, *The Prostitution Experience*: "When I think of my choices there were simply these: have men on and inside you, or continue to suffer homelessness and hunger. Take your pick. Make your 'choice.'"

We have decided to include empirical research from around the world of women who sell sex in many different contexts and for many different reasons. Clearly, there are socioeconomic influences at work for the women included in this review. These women will have made the choice to sell sex within some degree of constrained conditions, though some will have had more freedom of choice than others. Where we have drawn the line with regard to a deliberate decision to sell sex, is that we will exclude research on women who sell sex under overt coercion, such as sex trafficking or slavery, at least to the extent this is reported in the research.

We will start by exploring the wide variety of motivational factors why women start selling sex (Chap. 2). Next, the book will highlight some important sociocultural contexts surrounding the sale of sex that contribute to stress, and examine how women cope with these circumstances (Chap. 3). The heart of the book focuses on how selling sex relates to a host of mental health variables, which include potential precursors and outcomes of selling sex (Chap. 4). Next, the book examines the large literature on alcohol and drug use and abuse among women who sell sex (Chap. 5). Consistent with historical trends within the field of psychology, Chaps. 4 and 5 will place emphasis on mental health concerns. Despite the rise and popularity of the discipline of positive psychology, examination of positive topics such as meaningful personal strengths and qualities are rare in the study of selling sex, but will be included where available. Subsequently, the book will consider motivational factors for why women stop selling sex, what can make this change difficult, and what makes for successful transitions (Chap. 6). Having reviewed the research, we will offer implications for mental health professionals (Chap. 7) and provide a synthesis of the psychological knowledge about women who sell sex with directions for future research (Chap. 8).

Topics Excluded

As important as outlining the goals for the book, is delineating the boundaries of what will be covered. First, addressing psychological concepts relevant to women who choose to sell sex is not sufficient for offering a complete picture of how selling sex relates to overall wellbeing, which encompasses not only psychological, but also physical and spiritual domains. Addressing wholistic wellbeing would require a broader review of topics, as well as a deeper philosophical discussion about the body, use of the body, human sexuality, and how these topics relate to mind and spirit.

This book is not intended to offer conclusions about the overall merits or harms of selling sex or the morality of selling sex. This introduction to the psychological concepts related to selling sex is not equipped to endorse, indict, or even evaluate the larger institution of selling sex. What the book offers is a better understanding of some important psychological concepts relevant to women who sell sex. However, this is only one piece of a large and complex puzzle. For individuals hoping to develop or defend arguments for or against selling sex, understanding the extant psychology research may be important, but needs to be supplemented by other sources of knowledge relevant to arguments about the sale of sex, including empirical research from other disciplines, as well as theories and values from social, cultural, political, moral, and religious studies. Some topics in this book will overlap with topics of interest to other disciplines. However, the major contributions of other fields to understanding the sale of sex, such as the politics, economics, sociology, legality, and health issues involved in selling sex will be left to other books.

Definition of Selling Sex

Our definition of selling sex should be clarified. This book is focused specifically on private, in-person, consensual sex acts exchanged between a woman and a paying customer. Given this definition, activities such as pornography and erotic performances will not be covered. The emphasis will be primarily on selling sex for money. However, research has also focused on trading sex for other things of value, such as food, clothing, shelter, or drugs. This is sometimes referred to as transactional sex or indirect sex work. Using sex to obtain basic necessities is also called survival sex. Further, a topic of interest in recent popular culture has been young women using sex for things that go beyond basic necessities, such as to pay for higher education or to receive luxurious gifts (e.g., Motyl, 2013; Nayar, 2017). On closer consideration, there are many ways in which sex can become transactional in nature, ranging from the sugar baby whose sex partner pays her rent to the woman who does not want to say no because her date paid for dinner. Therefore, this concept can quickly become a fuzzy one. To maintain a clear focus, we will concentrate on the use of sex as an income-generating tool. Our review is inclusive of transactional sex only when this is combined with selling sex for money, such as when researchers group together trading sex for money *or* goods.

Populations Included in the Review

At the outset, some important distinctions should be made about the populations that will be examined. We will focus specifically on cisgender women. Men and transgendered individuals may have very different motivations, experiences, and mental health outcomes associated with selling sex (e.g., Burnette et al., 2008; Vanwesenbeeck, 2013). Therefore, we will mostly exclude studies in which analyses are conducted for men and women together. We make an exception for a few noteworthy studies that include a small percentage of men. In such cases, we will clearly highlight that the sample included some men.

In addition, as noted, we will not focus on research about victims of sex trafficking. Although the question of whether any or many women freely choose to sell sex is a contentious one, there is clear consensus that victims of sex trafficking have had no choice with regard to selling sex. As might be expected, the experiences and mental health correlates of trafficking victims differ from those of women who sell sex under other circumstances (e.g., Muftić & Finn, 2013). Unfortunately, how women first start selling sex is a variable that is not systematically assessed and reported in the research literature. This makes it likely that some proportion of study participants within the research reviewed in this book will have been trafficked or otherwise directly coerced into selling sex. Nevertheless, we will exclude research conducted explicitly among victims of trafficking. For similar reasons, research on children and youth will not be reviewed in this book, because minors are legally (and, one might argue, psychologically) not able to give informed consent to have sex. Therefore, exchanging money for sex with a minor falls outside of our definition of selling sex. Studies that include minors as participants will be excluded unless specifically noted, for example, in instances when study samples consist mostly of adults, but the age range begins slightly below adulthood. We will not use age of first involvement in the sale of sex as an exclusionary criterion, because this variable is not consistently reported in the research literature.

Nature of Research Included in the Review

Finally, this book is meant to offer a concise rather than a comprehensive review of psychology research on women selling sex. Our goal is to provide insight into what is known, how it has been studied, and what is still missing in the research literature. We will be most inclusive of research that examines women who sell sex in comparison to a peer group of women who do not sell sex, because research that focuses exclusively on women who sell sex is not able to account for the effects of other influential life factors. Therefore, we will be most comprehensive in reviewing comparative studies. In addition, we will focus more on research with quantitative rather than qualitative designs. A great deal of qualitative research has been conducted, and these studies provide rich detail. We will use qualitative findings for illustrative purposes, and will draw on qualitative work more extensively on topics where quantitative research is sparse. As a form of quality control, this book will favor peer-reviewed sources of research findings, meaning that the findings reviewed come primarily from journal articles, rather than from books, book chapters, dissertations, news articles, or other sources.

What's in a Name? The Terminology of Selling Sex

To date, the terms used in research to describe selling sex have contributed to both controversy and confusion. The two most common contenders are prostitution and sex work. The etymology of the term prostitute is the Latin *prostituere*, which comes from *pro*, meaning "before," and *statuere*, meaning "to set up" or "place." This term was originally used to describe a person who was publicly exposed or offered for sale. Although the root of this word is not necessarily derogatory, the early use included putting something to an unworthy use or dishonoring someone and exposing her to public shame. The primary definition for prostitution in the Oxford English Dictionary (2007) is value-neutral: "the practice or occupation of engaging in sexual activity with someone for payment;" however, some of the secondary definitions have a negative connotation, such as "licentiousness" and "lewdness."

Some have argued that the terms *prostitution* and *prostitute* are offensive, and therefore promote the use of the alternative terms *sex work* and *sex worker*. Proponents of the term sex work tend to argue that it lends dignity and professionalism to selling sex and that the term emphasizes that selling sex is a legitimate form of work. However, opponents of this term have argued that creating a polished image of selling sex serves only the sex industry, and not the women working in it. Along these lines, the Oxford English Dictionary (2008) notes that the term sex work is used both to diminish negative connotations and to evoke affinity with the sex industry. A particular limitation of the term sex work for the purpose of the current book is that it is broader in meaning, in that it includes commercial sexual services of any kind, such as pornography, exotic dancing, phone sex, internet webcam services, and other activities excluded from the current review.

The debate about terminology is often, at its core, a battle over how selling sex should be viewed within society and addressed by public policy. Advocates of the term sex work tend to emphasize legalization and acceptance of the choice to sell sex, whereas advocates of the term prostitution tend to emphasize the need to protect people from coercion and sex trafficking by abolishing commercial sex. What makes this controversy even more complex is that, in the absence of clear data, it is unclear how many women are represented by each side of the argument: vulnerable women who sell sex to survive versus middle class or elite women who have a free choice whether or not to sell sex.

These discussions are extremely important for many reasons, but are not the focus of this book. Divergent ideological stances about selling sex will be discussed briefly in the next section of this chapter as a foundation for understanding the various viewpoints undergirding research on women who sell sex. The point here is simply to provide a rationale for the terminology used in this book. Because the goal of this book is to review what can be learned from the empirical psychology literature about selling sex, without making an a priori argument about the meaning of selling sex, we will mostly use the behavioral description "selling sex" to avoid the value judgments and associations that may be linked to more commonly used terms. Our emphasis will be on selling sex as a behavior, rather than a personal descriptor or identity label. Therefore, we have chosen to use the more cumbersome "women who sell sex" over the alternative options of "prostitutes" or "sex workers."

Ideological Stances Toward Selling Sex

Common Ideologies

In approaching the research literature, it is important to acknowledge that theorists and researchers differ in their views of the causes, consequences, and responses to selling sex. On any topic of study, beliefs about the subject matter inform the formulation of research questions, hypotheses, and study methodologies. There are many different ideological stances to selling sex. We briefly consider three of the common ones, which equate selling sex to violence, legitimate work, and sexual freedom, respectively. Each of these stances is based on extensive theory from a variety of fields beyond psychology, including in particular feminism, but also philosophy, law, sociology, political science, and economics. Here, the goal is to briefly summarize some of the components of these theories in order to understand some of the perspectives that may underlie the research reviewed in this book. For more insight into the vigorous conversation around selling sex, see Spector's (2006) edited volume in which many of these ideas are debated from a philosophical perspective.

The view of selling sex as violence (e.g., Dworkin, 1997; Farley, 2003, 2004; Jeffreys, 2009; MacKinnon, 1993; Pateman, 1983, 1988, 1999; Raymond, 2013) often originates from the radical feminist perspective that selling sex involves the violent subordination of women by men, enabled by a patriarchal society in which women are viewed as sex objects. For example, Pateman (1983, p. 561, 1988) referred to selling sex as "one of the most graphic examples of men's domination of women." From this perspective, selling sex is equivalent to rape and sexual slavery, which, by their nature, cannot be voluntary. Also relevant to this ideological stance is the closely related idea that sexuality is intertwined with one's core identity, thereby making the sale of sex, which involves the most intimate parts of one's body, harmful not only to one's body, but also to one's self (Pateman, 1988). Consequently, those who equate selling sex with violence and harm advocate for abolishing prostitution. From this approach, selling sex is at its core always nonconsensual, even though some women submit to and collaborate with their social oppressors because this is less threatening than resisting. For these reasons, opponents of prostitution argue that characterizing selling sex as work or describing it in commercial or contractual terms is problematic (e.g., Pateman, 1983, 1988).

Those who view selling sex as legitimate work do not deny that coercion and sex trafficking exist, rather, they argue that these phenomena do not represent all cases of selling sex and that their existence does not negate the fact that there are many women who freely choose to sell sex. Thus, the argument is that voluntary and forced sale of sex are distinct and should not be confused with one another. Proponents of this perspective have included researchers (e.g., Weitzer, 2012), sex worker rights organizations such as COYOTE (see Jenness, 1990), labor unions representing sex workers (see Gall, 2007, 2016), and other organizations such as Anti-Slavery International (Bindman, 1997). They often aim to challenge the perception of women who sell sex as victims and replace this with an emphasis on agency. In this line of thinking, the sex industry is compared to conventional forms of labor. The idea is that selling sex is a simple "contractual relation in which services are traded" similar to those found in conventional service professions (Ericsson, 1980, p. 353). From this perspective, taking away women's rights to sell sex is to deny autonomy and self-determination for those who would choose to engage in this work. The assumption is made that women who sell sex should have labor rights similar to other workers and that important reforms may be needed with regard to the conditions under which sex is sold.

Finally, the view of selling sex as sexual freedom suggests that selling sex can be a positive expression of sexuality that can empower or otherwise benefit women (e.g., Bell, 1995, 2009; Queen, 1997). This perspective has been referred to as *pro-sex feminism*, *sex-positive feminism*, and *sex radical feminism* (Bernstein, 1999; Comte, 2014). Similar to the view that selling sex is violence, the view that selling sex is an expression of sexual freedom is grounded within feminist ideas about patriarchy creating an unhealthy sexual environment. However, rather than emphasizing the concepts of sexual objectification and exploitation, proponents of the view that selling sex represents sexual freedom emphasize that selling sex is an appropriate response to sexual repression and control. The thinking is that society controls women through stigmas, taboos, prejudices, and double standards surrounding sexuality. As such, selling sex can be viewed as a legitimate avenue for women to explore their sexuality and act against sexual guilt and inhibitions instilled by a patriarchal society.

Each of these ideologies about selling sex promotes different assumptions about the motivating factors for selling sex. For example, taking the perspective that selling sex is violence supports the idea that free consent to sell sex is highly unlikely or impossible, and that motivations to sell sex stem from external forces rather than internal motivators or choices. In contrast, the viewpoint that selling sex is legitimate work supports the notion that women are motivated to sell sex in the same fashion they are motivated to engage in any kind of work, when the ratio of benefits to costs is greatest for this work in comparison to other available work opportunities. When selling sex is viewed as a profession, consent can be thought of as being *more* explicit than in non-paid sexual encounters, because a priori agreements are made about the specific nature and length of sexual interaction. Finally, the perspective that selling sex represents sexual freedom promotes the idea that women are motivated to sell sex as a way to explore and express their sexual desires and emancipate themselves. From this perspective, it is possible that women find it intrinsically exciting and pleasurable to sell sex, which is in direct contrast to the notion that women say selling sex is a positive experience only as a way to cope with their *true* subjugation to external forces, an idea sometimes promoted by those who believe selling sex is violence.

Each of these ideologies about selling sex promotes different assumptions about the consequences of selling sex. The ideology that selling sex is equivalent to violence, rape, and sexual slavery naturally leads to the assumption that selling sex will result in post-traumatic stress and a host of other mental health problems for those subjected to this experience. In contrast, the ideology that selling sex is legitimate work does not presuppose that selling sex would cause mental health concerns; however, consideration is given to the social stigmatization and legal status of this work and the potentially associated negative consequences. Finally, the ideology that selling sex represents sexual freedom, with the notion that selling sex provides healthy sexual exploration and liberation from personal guilt and taboos, suggests that selling sex could result in positive psychological growth and greater well-being.

A final implication of the divergent ideologies about selling sex is that each of the viewpoints tends to promote different goals for responding to the sale of sex. Those who view selling sex as violence will fight for the abolition of the commercial sale of sex to protect those being harmed by it, taking the stance that selling sex harms women even if legalized or decriminalized (Farley, 2004; Raymond, 2004). They may also target the socioeconomic forces that contribute to women selling sex for survival purposes and prioritize creating viable alternative options for women. For additional abolition arguments, see Pateman (1988, 1999) and Raymond (2013). In contrast, those who maintain that selling sex is legitimate work often argue that selling sex should be decriminalized or legalized to give women an autonomous choice whether or not to engage in this activity. Those taking this perspective tend to focus on minimizing stigma and prejudice directed at women who sell sex and offering these women the respect of any type of worker. For reviews of legalization, see Sanders, O'Neil, and Pitcher (2018) or Weitzer (2012). Finally, of the three ideological stances, the argument that selling sex represents sexual freedom is the least commonly heard in public discourse, but similarly promotes the goals of decriminalization or legalization and destigmatization of selling sex. For example, Thompson (2000) argued that selling sex can be a tool of empowerment that allows women who choose it as a career to exercise personal power, economic freedom, and sexual autonomy, but that this can only occur if selling sex is decriminalized: "Only through a system of decriminalization can the social stigma associated with prostitution be erased, granting the freedom to choose prostitution as a respectable occupation" (pp. 217–128).

Even though those who adhere to different ideologies hold vastly different viewpoints with different implications for selling sex, there are points of commonality that are worth emphasizing, particularly with regard to their end goals. First, of importance to almost all those engaged with this topic is their care and concern for women's wellbeing and a desire for women to be empowered. All agree that consent is essential (whether or not they believe it is possible) and that human trafficking is abhorrent. Further, spokespeople on all sides maintain that what is needed is for women to have true alternatives. That is, even those who view selling sex as legitimate work do not necessarily believe that it is ideal work, or that it is suitable work for all, or even most, women.

Our Approach

Although we acknowledge that what is known about women selling sex is influenced, to a certain extent, by the ideological views of those researching this topic, we made efforts to take a neutral approach within our review of the literature. We include research on the basis of criteria about the research topic, sample, methodology, and publication type outlined in the section about the goals of this book, without favoring or excluding research on the basis of whether it supports any particular ideology about selling sex. That is not to say we claim to be personally value free with regard to a topic as controversial as selling sex. For example, some of our own values are guided by the belief in a mind–body-spirit connection. However, the purpose of this book is not to persuade or argue for an ideological perspective and we have made efforts to include research findings on the basis of objective inclusion criteria rather than personal convictions.

We approach this project on the basis of our professional interests and training in the fields of Clinical Psychology (EKM) and Industrial/Organizational Psychology and Health Management (BEP). My (EKM) interest in the topic was first sparked while growing up in the Netherlands at a time in which there were ongoing discussions surrounding the tolerance and then legalization of prostitution. For a period of time, the government's stance was that selling sex was a job like any other, meaning it was advertised by employment agencies and sex workers registered with the chamber of commerce, paid taxes, and joined trade unions. Many of these circumstances remain the same, though the official stance has shifted to acknowledge that, although selling sex is a job, it is not a job *like any other*. This book explores some of the potentially unique characteristics of selling sex.

In the past decade, I (EKM) have had conversations about selling sex in numerous European countries with historians of prostitution, prostitution educators, political activists, physicians working in public health with the World Health Organization and Joint United Nations Programme on HIV/AIDS, counter-trafficking program and project officers with the International Organization for Migration, police force program coordinators and officers on prostitution task forces, and women currently and formerly selling sex. In recent years, we (EKM and BEP) have researched selling sex in the Netherlands, talking with a wide variety of women selling sex, venue managers, and task force police officers throughout the country.

Based on these experiences and our review of the literature, we believe empirical data regarding the lived experiences of women who sell sex can be used (and misused) in support of each of the three discussed ideologies of selling sex. We believe many women are forced or coerced into selling sex, many become involved for financial reasons (including out of desperation or out of a desire to earn money in this way), some seek it for liberation and excitement, and many experience a combination of motivational factors. We believe a wide range of psychological correlates of selling sex exists precisely because of the diversity among women who sell sex and their myriad reasons for doing so. In writing this book, we emphasize that the interrelationships between selling sex and potential precursors and outcomes are often complex and open to interpretation. These complexities will be points of discussion in the book, to allow readers to have a more nuanced understanding of the existing literature on women who sell sex.

Methodological Considerations in the Empirical Research on Women Who Sell Sex

Before reviewing what the empirical psychology literature has to contribute to an understanding of the motivating factors and psychological correlates of selling sex, it is important to have some overarching insight into the nature of the research that has been conducted and how the available data may constrain conclusions. Relevant methodological considerations include how selling sex has been defined and assessed, the nature of the groups that have been studied, and the type of information that has been gathered. We will briefly discuss each of these issues.

Operational Definitions

There are a number of different ways in which selling sex is operationally defined in the research literature. We have already noted that this book will focus primarily on women who sell sex for money, but will also include some research on women who trade sex for goods when the results are combined with selling sex for money. The goods most often assessed in the literature include food, clothes, housing, drugs, and alcohol. Thus, it is important to realize that research outcomes may differ for women who accept different types of payment for sex. For example, a woman who sells sex for money may be in a very different life situation than a woman who trades sex for a place to stay or for drugs. Therefore, different research findings across studies may relate to the way that selling sex was operationalized.

There are additional differences across studies in the way selling sex is measured. For example, some studies focus on participants who have ever been paid for sex. Studies that take such a lifetime history approach place anyone who has ever accepted payment for sex in a sex selling group and everyone else in a comparison group. Another approach is to assess whether women are currently active in selling sex or not, for example, by asking whether they have accepted payment for sex within the previous month, six months, or year. Though rarer, some researchers have focused only on women who sell sex on a regular basis, defining this as selling sex at least once per week. It is important to keep in mind that asking different questions leads to different answers. Thus, the variety of ways in which selling sex is assessed within the research literature is bound to lead to nuances within the research results.

Samples

To better understand the literature base, it is also critical to reflect on the nature of the samples that have been studied. The legal and social status of selling sex in many countries has serious implication for research. Because selling sex is illegal and/or stigmatized in many places, it becomes difficult to have an accurate picture of the full population of women who sell sex. Furthermore, women who can be identified and recruited may not participate because of privacy concerns.

The fact that, in many locations, women who sell sex are a *hidden population* (Cusick, Kinnell, Brooks-Gordon, & Campbell, 2009) makes it unlikely that researchers are able to recruit anything close to a representative sample. This is complicated by the fact that the sale of sex occurs in many different settings. Often, selling sex in the street, or street-level work, is used to refer to transactions that originate outdoors, and take place in parks, cars, motels, at truck stops, or in crack houses. Selling sex indoors generally refers to working in a brothel, club, massage parlor, or from home. Thus far, the samples of women that have been studied have most commonly consisted of those who are the most visible and accessible. In countries where prostitution is illegal, these are typically women who are working on the streets, incarcerated, or in substance abuse or crisis treatment. This means a fair amount of research on women who sell sex has included samples with high prevalence rates of substance abuse and experiences of violence. Indoor sale of sex, which represents the majority form of selling sex in many countries, has only more recently been the target of research (O'Doherty, 2011). It is important to realize that the activity of selling sex is multifaceted and presents in many different forms. Therefore, the research findings of one group of women do not necessarily generalize to other groups of women, especially those who find themselves in different kinds of working conditions. Thus, in trying to understand women who sell sex, it is important to take particular caution when attempting to generalize research findings beyond the women studied.

Along similar lines, it is important to remember that data that describe a group do not necessarily describe any particular individual within that group. Quantitative research on groups of women who sell sex are often based on analyses of mean scores on variables of interest; however, there may be a great deal of variance within the group. Therefore, it is not possible to use research findings to make assumptions about any given woman who sells sex. This is particularly important to keep in mind when using research findings to inform clinical work (see Chap. 7).

In addition, it is important to consider the nature of comparison samples that have been assessed in research. Some studies have compared samples of women who sell sex to same-aged women from the general population. This does not account for the many differences that exist between these two groups. As noted, many researchers have studied samples of women who sell sex who are in vulnerable life situations. Comparing these groups to women in the general population does not account for the many challenges and problems faced by the women who sell sex. Other studies have taken greater care to find more similar comparison groups, sometimes matching the groups on the basis of a host of demographic and background factors. Most research has also statistically controlled for important demographic differences between the groups being compared, such as race, ethnicity, socioeconomic status, and level of education. This offers a bit more confidence that research findings are not attributable to other life differences that exist between women who do and do not sell sex; however, studies have differed in the number of variables they have controlled, and only some of the studies have considered important factors beyond basic demographics, such as substance abuse and history of violence.

The Nature of the Data

Another important methodological topic is the nature of the information collected. Although some studies base analyses on objective data such as arrest records or mental health diagnoses, the vast majority of studies utilize self-report data. For any population studied in the field of psychology, questions exist regarding the accuracy of information that is reported. Gathering accurate information from research participants requires that participants have insight into the topics being assessed and are able to recall information correctly. Furthermore, given the sensitivity of the topic, getting accurate information also depends on the extent to which women are willing to share personal information openly and honestly. Research examining the accuracy of self-report data from women who sell sex is rare. However, the studies that have evaluated this seem to indicate that the information gained is reasonably reliable. For example, in one study examining pathways into selling sex, women were interviewed about their life histories twice, a year apart (Potterat, Rothenberg, Muth, Darrow, & Phillips-Plummer, 1998). This indicated that the women reported the timing of life events fairly consistently, with 70% of the women giving answers that were within one year of their original estimates and 84% giving answers that were within two years of their original answers. This was within the context of a sample among which substance abuse was common, which may have negatively impacted memory. Similar rates of agreement have been found by studies administering written surveys about selling sex at two different points in time (e.g., a test–retest reliability coefficient of 0.74 was found by Popoola, 2013). Thus, the information gained by self-report, whether via interviews or written surveys, is far from perfect, but seems reliable enough to warrant use in research.

Regardless of whether the data collected are objective or subjective in nature, all studies about selling sex will be correlational in nature. It should be clear that experimental research in which some women are randomly assigned to sell sex is neither feasible nor ethical. Therefore, causality cannot be established between selling sex and potential predictors or outcomes. The best approximations come from longitudinal studies that collect data at multiple points in time, especially prospective studies that start following women before their first encounter with commercial sex. This type of research can provide insight into the time ordering of variables and rule out some of the potential confounds that would otherwise be present. Unfortunately, this type of research is exceedingly rare when it comes to women who sell sex.

Conclusions

What should be clear from the discussion of the themes in the existing research on women who sell sex is that the phenomenon of selling sex is extremely diverse, and therefore, psychological predictors and outcomes of selling sex are likely to differ as a function of the definitions used, the samples studied, and the nature of the data. For this reason, a book on the psychology of selling sex calls for a nuanced rather than a general discussion of this topic. With this in mind, let's turn to the research that explores why women first start selling sex.

References

Bell, S. (1995). *Whore carnival*. New York: Autonomedia.

Bell, K. J. (2009). A feminists argument on how sex work can benefit women. *Inquiries Journal/Student Pulse, 1*(11).

Bernstein, E. (1999). What's wrong with prostitution? What's right with sex work? Comparing markets in female sexual labor. *Hastings Women's Law Journal, 10,* 91–117.

Bindman, J. (1997). Redefining prostitution as sex work on the international agenda. *Anti-Slavery International*. Retrieved July 30, 2018, from https://walnet.org/csis/papers/redefining.html.

Burnette, M. L., Lucas, E., Ilgen, M., Frayne, S. M., Mayo, J., & Weitlauf, J. C. (2008). Prevalence and health correlates of prostitution among patients entering treatment for substance use disorders. *Archives of General Psychiatry, 65,* 337–344. https://doi.org/10.1001/archpsyc.65.3.337

Comte, J. (2014). Decriminalization of sex work: Feminist discourses. *Sexuality & Culture, 18,* 196–217. https://doi.org/10.1007/s12119-013-9174-5

Cusick, L., Kinnell, H., Brooks-Gordon, B., & Campbell, R. (2009). Wild guesses and conflated meanings? Estimating the size of the sex worker population in Britain. *Critical Social Policy, 29,* 703–719. https://doi.org/10.1177/0261018309341906

Dworkin, A. (1997). *Life and death: Unapologetic writings on the continuing war against women*. New York: Free Press.

Ericsson, L. O. (1980). Charges against prostitution: An attempt at a philosophical assessment. *Ethics, 90,* 335–366.

Farley, M. (2003). Prostitution and the invisibility of harm. *Women & Therapy, 26,* 247–280. https://doi.org/10.1300/J015v26n03_06

Farley, M. (2004). "Bad for the body, bad for the heart": Prostitution harms women even if legalized or decriminalized. *Violence Against Women, 10,* 1087–1125. https://doi.org/10.1177/1077801204268607

Gall, G. (2007). Sex worker unionisation: An exploratory study of emerging collective organisation. *Industrial Relations Journal, 38,* 70–88. https://doi.org/10.1111/j.1468-2338.2007.00436.x

Gall, G. (2016). *Sex worker unionisation: Global developments, challenges, and possibilities*. Basingstoke, UK: Palgrave Macmillan.

Jenness, V. (1990). From sex as sin to sex as work: COYOTE and the reorganization of prostitution as social problem. *Social Problems, 37,* 403–420. https://doi.org/10.2307/800751

Jeffreys, S. (2009). *The industrial vagina: The political economy of the global sex trade*. London: Routledge.

MacKinnon, C. (1993). Prostitution and civil rights. *Michigan Journal of Gender & Law, 1,* 13–31.

Moran, R. (2012, February 8). A personal refutation of the concept of 'choice'. Blog Post. Retrieved from https://theprostitutionexperience.com/?p=10.

Motyl, J. (2013). Trading sex for college tuition: How sugar daddy dating sites may be sugar coating prostitution. *Penn State Law Review, 117,* 927–957.

Muftić, L. R., & Finn, M. A. (2013). Health outcomes among women trafficked for sex in the United States. *Journal of Interpersonal Violence, 28,* 1859–1885. https://doi.org/10.1177/0886260512469102

Nayar, K. I. (2017). Sweetening the deal: Dating for compensation in the digital age. *Journal of Gender Studies, 27,* 335–346. https://doi.org/10.1080/09589236.2016.1273101

O'Doherty, T. (2011). Victimization in Off-street sex industry work. *Violence Against Women, 17,* 944–963. https://doi.org/10.1177/1077801211412917

Pateman, C. (1983). Defending prostitution: Charges against Ericsson. *Ethics, 93,* 561–565.

Pateman, C. (1988). *The sexual contract*. Stanford, CA: Stanford University Press.

Pateman, C. (1999). What wrong with prostitution? *Women's Studies Quarterly, 27,* 53–64.

Popoola, B. I. (2013). Occupational hazards and coping strategies of sex workers in southwestern Nigeria. *Health Care for Women International, 34,* 139–149. https://doi.org/10.1080/07399332.2011.646366

Potterat, J. J., Rothenberg, R. B., Muth, S. Q., Darrow, W. W., & Phillips-Plummer, L. (1998). Pathways to prostitution: The chronology of sexual and drug abuse milestones. *Journal of Sex Research, 35,* 333–340. https://doi.org/10.1080/00224499809551951

Prostitution. (2007, June). *The Oxford English dictionary* (3rd edn.). Retrieved from www.oed.com/view/Entry/153086.

Queen, C. (1997). *Real live nude girl: Chronicles of sex-positive culture.* San Francisco, CA: Cleis Press.

Raymond, J. G. (2004). Ten reasons for not legalizing prostitution and a legal response to the demand for prostitution. *Journal of Trauma Practice, 2,* 315–332. https://doi.org/10.1300/J189v02n03_17

Raymond, J. G. (2013). *Not a choice, not a job: Exposing the myths about the prostitution trade.* Washington, DC: Potomac Books.

Sanders, T., O'Neill, M., & Pitcher, J. (2018). *Prostitution: Sex work, policy and politics* (2nd ed.). London: Sage.

Sex Work. (2008, December). *The Oxford English dictionary* (3rd ed.). Retrieved from https://www.oed.com/view/Entry/176989.

Spector, J. (Ed.). (2006). *Prostitution and pornography: Philosophical debate about the sex industry.* Stanford, CA: Stanford University Press.

Thompson, S. E. (2000). Prostitution—A choice ignored. *Women's Rights Law Reporter, 21,* 217–247.

Vanwesenbeeck, I. (2013). Prostitution push and pull: Male and female perspectives. *Journal of Sex Research, 50,* 11–16. https://doi.org/10.1080/00224499.2012.696285

Weitzer, R. (2010). Sex work: Paradigms and policies. In R. Weitzer (Ed.), *Sex for sale: Prostitution, pornography, and the sex industry* (2nd ed., pp. 1–43). New York: Routledge.

Weitzer, R. (2012). *Legalizing prostitution: From illicit vice to lawful business.* New York: New York University Press.

Chapter 2
Motivations for Selling Sex

Given the physically intimate nature of sex and the fact that selling sex is often considered *dirty work* (see Chap. 3), one might wonder what factors influence women to have sex for money. This chapter focuses on increasing understanding about why and how women first start selling sex. As noted in the previous chapter, one prevalent ideology is that women, in fact, do not freely choose to sell sex, but are coerced by external factors. These external factors can be direct factors, such as pimps or brothel owners, or indirect factors, such as sex discrimination, poverty, lack of education, or jobs that don't pay a living wage (e.g., Farley, 2006). Some who are vocally opposed to women selling sex argue that the conditions that would make genuine consent possible are absent, including physical safety, equal power with customers, and access to alternative options (Farley et al., 2003; MacKinnon, 1993; Raymond, 2013).

Despite some viewing only external factors as the driving forces behind women selling sex, this chapter will review psychological research being inclusive of both external influences *and* free will factors associated with starting to sell sex from the vantage point of the individual woman. We further acknowledge that the sociopolitical and economic factors that influence women to sell sex are extremely important to consider; however, given that this book is focused on the *psychology* of sexual commerce, more macro level factors will be left to reviews conducted from other disciplinary perspectives, such as sociology, political science, economics, and criminology. The research reviewed in this chapter draws on three primary sources: self-reports from women describing why they started selling sex, comparative research examining differences between women who do and do not sell sex, and clinical theories about why women sell sex.

Given that the most common source of information on this topic is what women say motivated them to sell sex, it's relevant to note that some researchers have raised concern about whether descriptions from women who sell sex can be interpreted as straightforward accounts of reality (e.g., Vanwesenbeeck, 2001; Weatherall & Priestley, 2001). For example, women describing the experience of feeling powerful or powerless in their choice to sell sex may not reflect true power or powerlessness.

E. Krumrei Mancuso and B. E. Postlethwaite, *Women Who Sell Sex*,
https://doi.org/10.1007/978-3-030-47027-2_2

In addition, women's responses to interviews and surveys may be interpreted by researchers in a way that reflects biases or lack of understanding. We consider these potential concerns to be valid, but no different than the concerns about self-reported research on other topics. Psychological research often relies heavily on self-reported information. Self-reports are useful only to the extent that individuals have insight into the topics being asked about, can remember information accurately, and are willing to share information honestly. Data of all kinds are subject to potential biases from participants and researchers. Despite these concerns, we continue to see value in listening to the factors women describe as having contributed to their choice to sell sex.

Financial Factors

Economic gain is a very commonly cited motivational factor for women who sell sex. This ranges from those who are homeless, widowed, or fleeing from abuse who start selling sex to sustain basic needs (e.g., Goldenberg, Engstrom, Rolon, Silverman, & Strathdee, 2013; Harding & Hamilton, 2009; Suresh, Furr, & Srikrishnan, 2009; Thappa, Singh, & Kaimal, 2007) to middle-class women who choose to sell sex to cover their living expenses or to afford luxuries (e.g., Bernstein, 2007; Krumrei-Mancuso, 2017; Sanders, 2002).

A Taiwanese study exploring why women[1] sell sex found that almost all of the participants provided financial reasons (McCaghy, & Hou, 1994). These included providing financial assistance to parents (34% of the sample), paying off personal or spousal debt (29% of the sample), desiring an easy life, materialism, or improved status (17% of the sample), and economic survival after escaping negative family or marriage situations (9% of the sample). In a study of women selling sex in licensed brothels in Victoria, Australia, women also reported selling sex primarily for financial gain, with 69% of women citing "a need for money" and 76% "having a particular financial goal in mind" (Bilardi et al., 2011, p. 118). Platt et al. (2011) examined financial motivations for selling sex among women who worked indoors in London. Nearly half of the women identified paying for household expenses or supporting family as the main financial reason for selling sex. For other women, the primary motivation included financing studies or savings (23.4%), funding social life (12.5%), and drugs (4%). Of note is the overlap between finances and many other motivational factors reviewed in this chapter, including relational influences, substance abuse, and selling sex as a rational choice.

---

[1]The participants in this study were mostly adults, however, the age range started at 16 years.

Relational Influences

As noted in Chap. 1, this book does not focus on women who are trafficked or otherwise forced into selling sex. Yet, there are many other ways women can be more subtly coerced or otherwise influenced to sell sex by people they are in relationship with. It is well known that pimps exert coercive power, but it is important to emphasize that this can take many forms. Some women describe starting to sell sex on the basis of encouragement or coercion from a violent man who vacillates between the roles of boyfriend, drug dealer, and pimp (e.g., DeHart, Lynch, Belknap, Dass-Brailsford, & Green, 2014). Other times, a subtler influence is at work. A man may gently win the love and trust of a woman through attention and gifts and then, with or without a premeditated plan, convince her to sell sex for his monetary gain. In the Netherlands, this has been described as a *loverboy* (Bovenkerk & van San, 2011).

Aside from pimps/loverboys, family members are also a common relational influence toward selling sex in many countries. Family impoverishment can make a woman feel obligated to earn money by selling sex to better the lives of her parents, siblings, or children. In some cultural settings, selling sex is viewed as an income-generating opportunity and advancement strategy for a family (e.g., Rael, 2015). Selling sex to support one's family of origin is most common among cultures where a sense of familial obligation is a strong influence in women's lives (e.g., McCaghy, & Hou, 1994). In contrast to selling sex to support one's family, some women start selling sex to escape dysfunctional homes, marriage problems, or abuse (e.g., Abramovich, 2005; McCaghy, & Hou, 1994; Suresh et al., 2009).

Qualitative work has indicated that peer influence is also a major motivational factor in the decision to sell sex (Rosen & Venkatesh, 2008). In locations where selling sex is common, women learn at a young age about this option as they encounter other women who view it as an acceptable way to earn money. These factors make it more likely that women will view selling sex as a feasible employment choice.

Substance Abuse

Addiction can drive women to sell sex to acquire the necessary funds to purchase drugs or it can drive them to trade sex directly for drugs. In a number of studies, a majority of women reported they began selling sex as a means of funding their substance addictions (e.g., Cobbina & Oselin, 2011; Morris et al., 2013; Murphy, 2010; Roxburgh, Degenhardt, & Copeland, 2006). However, even in these cases, drugs may be only one of multiple reasons for starting to sell sex. For example, in a study from Australia, 52% of women reported that they sold sex to pay for drugs, but only 7% reported that drugs were the *only* reason they sold sex (Roxburgh et al., 2006).

In addition, the rates of substance abuse as a motivating factor for selling sex differ depending on a woman's context. For example, in a study of women selling sex in

London, Platt et al. (2011) found that 10% of participants born in the UK identified paying for drugs as their main financial reason for selling sex, whereas none of the participants from Eastern Europe or the Former Soviet Union identified drugs as their main financial reason for selling sex. The complex links between selling sex and substance addictions are discussed in more detail in Chap. 5.

Personal Interest

Personal interest can be another motivational factor for selling sex. Those who have a personal interest in selling sex desire to engage in this activity for its own sake rather than to gain something or to fulfill some other purpose. Meaning, some women start selling sex because they believe they will enjoy doing so. A number of studies have documented that selling sex can be desirable work for women. Research from Australia has indicated that women who sell sex have similar or higher levels of satisfaction with their work than women in other professions (Bilardi et al., 2011; Seib, Dunne, Fischer, & Najman, 2012). In one study, women who sold sex reported comparable or better satisfaction with their work compared to women in more traditional work sectors (Seib et al., 2012). The vast majority of these women who sold sex agreed that their work was varied and interesting (81%) and more than three-quarters agreed that it lived up to their expectations (78%). A little less than two-thirds of the women indicated they would choose a similar job if they had it to do over again (63%). In addition, a substantial minority of the women who sold sex indicated that their work was a major source of satisfaction in their lives (44%). Moreover, levels of satisfaction with selling sex as a job were unrelated to the amount of money earned in this study.

In another Australian study, women identified the jobs they would be most likely to do if they did not sell sex, and the researchers compared levels of job satisfaction between the women who sold sex and Australian women working in the jobs identified to be the most likely alternatives (Bilardi et al., 2011). Compared to Australian women in their most likely alternative jobs, 64% of women who sold sex reported the same or higher median levels of job satisfaction for total pay, 62% of women who sold sex reported the same or higher median levels of job satisfaction for hours worked, and 66% of women who sold sex reported the same or higher median levels of job satisfaction for the flexibility of balancing work and life commitments. Interestingly, compared to Australian women in their most likely alternative jobs, 47% of women who sold sex reported at least the same or higher median level of overall job satisfaction and 38% of the women who sold sex had the same or higher level of satisfaction with the work itself. In fact, 25% of women who sold sex had *higher* median levels of overall job satisfaction and 19% of women who sold sex had *higher* median levels of satisfaction with the work itself compared to Australian women in their most likely alternative jobs. Thus, while women who sell sex rate their satisfaction with their work high primarily for financial reasons, a minority of women who sell sex seem to be relatively satisfied with the work itself, and may prefer it over other work they could do. That said, in the same study, Billardi and colleagues found that women who sold sex were significantly *less likely* than Australian women to be satisfied or completely satisfied with regard to their financial situation, employment conditions, feelings of safety, feeling a part of their community, health, and life overall.

Thus far, we have systematically excluded research results in which the findings of men and women who sell sex are combined, however, we make an exception here to note the early findings of a multi-year study of 240 individuals (81.7% women) who used the internet to sell sex in the UK, recruited from online safety organization (Sanders, Connelly, & King, 2016). The sample consisted primarily of White, British, educated females. Although participants acknowledged selling sex was unpredictable (91% of sample), substantial percentages of the sample described their work using positive terms such as flexible (91%), fun (66%), rewarding (56%), skillful (53%), stimulating (45%), and empowering (50%), rather than using negative terms such as dehumanizing (15%) or exploitative (14%). Unfortunately, this study did not present a gender break-down of the results, so it is unclear to what extent the smaller portion of men and transgender individuals in the sample contributed to these overall numbers.

Although these quantitative studies from Australia and the UK are likely not representative of most women who sell sex throughout the world, this research illustrates that there are women who are quite satisfied with selling sex as a job. Smaller, qualitative studies have explored in more detail the underlying reasons why women may enjoy selling sex. It's not uncommon for women selling sex in certain settings to say they value the social aspect of their work, such as getting to meet interesting people, make social connections, and develop close relationships with regular customers (e.g., Rosen & Venkatesh, 2008). This theme is further illustrated in the case examples provided in this chapter (Text Box 2.1). In addition, some women report a sense of mastery, empowerment, pride, or self-worth derived from earning money by selling sex (Rosen & Venkatesh, 2008; Williamson & Folaron, 2003). For example, among women in Thailand, sending financial contributions to family members, earned by selling sex, is associated with optimism because of feelings of pride about helping one's family to have better living conditions (Ariyabuddhiphongs & Li, 2012). Such research illustrates how financial, relational, and personal satisfaction factors work together to motivate the activity of selling sex.

Text Box 2.1 Qualitative Interviews with Women Arguing for Their Desire to Sell Sex: The Cases of Anka and Jasmijn

Overview

The majority of research on selling sex describes motivational factors associated with distress or need. However, as highlighted in this chapter, some women choose to sell sex out of personal interest and desire. Here, descriptions of two qualitative interviews are provided to illustrate what this might look like. The interviews were conducted with two Dutch women selling sex legally in the Netherlands. The women emphasized that they experienced selling sex as meaningful and that it contributed to their wellbeing.

Method

The interviewed women reached out to the primary author following participation in a quantitative study conducted in the Netherlands (Krumrei-Mancuso, 2017), wanting their voices to be heard in more detail. They were subsequently interviewed for the purpose of this book. The interviews took place in Dutch. Pseudonyms are used to protect the women's privacy.

Case 1: Anka

At the time of the interview, Anka was 26 years old, single, and did not have any children. She first sold sex in her home and subsequently transitioned to a window brothel, where she worked part-time at the time of the interview. Her number of customers and therefore her income from selling sex was unpredictable from week to week. She had vocational training and worked in the hospitality industry for the remainder of her income, but described looking forward to selling sex much more than her other job. In follow-up conversations after the interview, Anka happily reported that she had quit her other job and started selling sex fulltime.

Motivation to sell sex

Anka described her conviction that the world revolves around power, sex, and money, and that everyone has to figure out how to maintain themselves in that reality. She described that she had always had an interest in selling sex, and had a sense as a young person that she would become a prostitute one day. At the age of 17, she daydreamed about standing behind a window.

Her first experience with selling sex was planned together with her boyfriend at the time; they arranged to have customers come to their home. Her boyfriend felt jealous, but went along with her selling sex because he also benefitted from the money. Because of the safety risks involved in having people come to her home, Anka chose to start working behind a window.

Anka first seriously considered selling sex on the basis of financial need, but she also viewed selling sex as an excuse for something exciting in her life. Interestingly, Anka described selling sex as an alternative to riskier ways of seeking excitement: "The money is a great perk, but it's especially the excitement of the work that motivates me. By selling sex I don't have to seek excitement in other ways that may put me in dangerous situations." What she especially liked about selling sex was that she got to pretend to be someone else, someone she couldn't be in real life.

In the interview, Anka touched on a number of topics common to the literature on the predictors of selling sex (see this chapter and Chap. 4). Anka was raped twice in her youth, experienced depression, and had been diagnosed with borderline personality disorder. There were times in her life she drank excessively and was suicidal. Yet, Anka did not view any of these factors as predictors of her selling sex. She had to learn to navigate her traumas and mental health conditions and intentionally waited until she was emotionally stable before she started selling sex. Anka argued that even women who have been sexually abused should have the choice of whether they want to sell sex or not. She described that depression runs in her family, and was not a trigger nor a result of selling sex in her case. In her view, some women may become depressed from selling sex, but she believed that is no different than becoming depressed from any type of work, like joining the army or having an office job.

Consequences of Selling Sex

Selling sex impacted Anka's life on individual, interpersonal, and social levels. On an individual level, Anka described her work as both physically and emotionally challenging. On her first day working at the window brothel, she saw 13 customers in 14 h. Afterwards, she couldn't ride her bike home because she had such sore muscles.

Her greatest emotional challenge was that working with her body could make it difficult to stay professional. She explained that selling sex is not equivalent to making love. She constantly had to remind herself what real sex was, and that she couldn't give this to customers. Otherwise, she was afraid selling sex would become too large a part of her life and that she would become a nymphomaniac. This view that the sex exchange with a customer is not true sex and has to be separated from what occurs with a romantic partner has been observed in other interviews with women who sell sex, as well (e.g., Oerton & Phoenix, 2001; Sanders, 2002).

Anka described various psychological mechanisms she developed to protect herself while working. She would focus her thoughts on other things to maintain peace and create mental distance while selling sex, mundane things, like her shopping list. Anka would also stick to the time limit and prohibit certain actions, like kissing. Otherwise, the relationship between herself and her customers could become ambiguous. When Anka would feel uncomfortable or attracted to a customer, she would delve further into a persona in order to distance herself. She described realizing the potential risk that she might lose herself in her role. The other women, window brothel administrators, and customers all called her by her character name. This would cause her real name to sound strange to her sometimes. She took measures to separate her persona when selling sex from the rest of her life. For example, she used a different perfume when working than in daily life. She also stored her work clothes in an unused room in her house, so that she wouldn't see them in her daily life. This type of behavior reflects what has been described as a double self or a second persona that women who sell sex have been known to use as a protective mechanism that creates the distance required to ward of personal emotions or sexual interest in customers (Bernstein, 2007; Sanders, 2005).[2] Interestingly, Anka described that on days she couldn't sell sex, she might want to be around her work clothes, to smell them and have a moment to escape into a memory of selling sex for a brief intermingling of her two lives.

On an interpersonal level, the consequences of selling sex included strained relationships in Anka's life. Despite selling sex being a huge part of her life, only three people in her life knew that she sold sex. Her bond with those she had told grew tremendously, because she was able to be herself fully in these relationships. But she kept this part of her life a secret from everyone else. She described this as the hardest aspect of her work, that she couldn't discuss it with people. She indicated that even if society would accept her choice, she would never tell her father and grandfather. This is consistent with the literature, which indicates that many women maintain secrecy about their selling sex in order to avoid being despised (Comte, 2014). It is a common observation in interviews with women who sell sex that their relationships are complicated or compromised by their selling sex (e.g., Oerton & Phoenix, 2001; Warr & Pyett, 1999). Because selling sex was such a large part of Anka's life, she was constantly lying to her close friends. This resulted in her living a double life. It was difficult to her that she could not share something she experienced as such a big aspect of who she was. She liked to talk about her work, but felt limited in where she could do so because others didn't view it as good work.

Although her selling sex strained most of her preexisting relationships due to her secrecy, Anka found new relationships through her work. She described having pleasant interactions with the other women who rented window rooms near her. They would sit in their rooms with the internal doors open, so that they could chat with each other while waiting for customers. They talked about what they had in common, their shared experiences, their customers, and their motivations for selling sex. Anka described learning a lot from the other women about life. She spoke fondly of a 40-year old woman who took her under her wing and shared tips with her.

Anka also described having positive interactions with the administrators of the window brothel. She described them as kind and concerned for the women, often checking into see how they were doing. They would provide a meal for her every Friday, and always walked her to her car after a shift, because she would be carrying cash. She also described having a lot of nice customers. She would look forward to them coming back. Some of them would bring her food or small gifts. She described how pleasant it was that these customers, who really didn't know her, did nice things for her.

However, outside of her work setting, Anka faced social stigma about her work. Anka felt that people judged her, assuming she was dumb and didn't use her brains. She described how exposed she felt when going to the chamber of commerce to register herself as a sex worker. She felt vulnerable when having to report how many customers she would have and how much money she would make. Anka was passionate about the fact that the social perceptions about women who sell sex are inaccurate. She believed selling sex requires business skills, people skills, and task-specific skills. She did not view selling sex as selling her body, but as selling an illusion. Putting on her makeup put her in a new role. She would sell the illusion that each man was her favorite customer or that she was in love, while in reality she kept a distance from her customers. She described the complexity of this craft. This is consistent with some reviews of research indicating that women who sell sex are selling a product, one they often view as a performance, whether that be a sexual fantasy, girlfriend experience, sexual arousal, stimulation, or satisfaction (Comte, 2014).

Although less common, Anka encountered some people who accepted her choice. She described these people as being curious and asking a lot of questions. She considered this a favorable social response.

Agency: Victims or willing workers?

Anka described that those who knew about her choice couldn't understand that she would voluntarily sell sex. This was consistent with the general social perception Anka encountered: people assumed she did not truly want to sell sex. However, she was adamant that she sold sex by choice, as evidenced by the time she had invested in pursuing this option. It took months of research and administrative tasks to work legally. She had to learn how to become an independent entrepreneur, register with the chamber of commerce and tax authorities, and find a window to rent. Once working, she had to go to the community health services every three months for testing.

Anka understood that not all women are cut out for selling sex. But she argued that this should not preclude those who truly want to do so from having the opportunity. However, Anka's experience was complex and enigmatic. She described that she enjoyed selling sex and looked forward to going to work. Yet, she also described days where she would wonder what she was doing. She described what she called the "mirror feeling" in which she would see herself in the mirror engaged in a sex act and experience a moment of clarity in which she would feel she had made a ridiculous choice. This paradox is not unique to Anka. Many women who sell sex are torn between feelings of pride and feelings of guilt regarding their work (Comte, 2014).

Empowerment versus exploitation

Anka realized some view selling sex as a form of violence, but she did not understand this perception. She would feel judged by the social perception that women who sell sex were poor or had been abused. She did not believe she fit this stereotype. Anka said she chose to sell sex because it was a good fit for her. She described that she really enjoyed sex; even sex with customers was enjoyable to her. She would look forward to the days she was in her window room. Her father always told her she should make a career out of her hobby, and that is what she did by selling sex.

Anka considered the money she received by selling sex to be a nice bonus on top of the enjoyment of the work. For example, she was proud that she was able to buy her own car. But Anka was adamant that selling sex was not primarily about the money for her. She described many positive aspects of selling sex in her life. It allowed her to express herself. It gave her an outlet to be herself in a way that nothing else did. She described the paradox of getting to be fully herself while also getting to choose when to take on the persona of someone else. In addition, selling sex served a protective mechanism in her life. She had always had the tendency to seek excitement, which at times caused problems for her. She would often bring men home whom she met in her night life. Selling sex became her way to fulfill her desire for excitement through work, which resulted in her private life becoming much calmer.

Anka said she did not have an inferiority complex, contrary to social perceptions about women who sell sex. She described that selling sex required a strong sense of self. Out of 10 men who would look at her in the window, only one would come in. Fortunately, she did not feel dependent on the approval of these men, and therefore would not feel bad about herself when a man did not pick her. On the other hand, she would experience a sense of fulfillment when a customer picked her out of the group of 10–12 women working in her window brothel. She viewed it as a compliment when a man chose her or when a man would return again.

Anka did not view selling sex as oppressive. She set her own limits as to what she would do for money. If potential customers were obnoxious, denigrating, or drunk, she wouldn't let them in. Outside of those situations, she was not too picky, she said; she had to make money, after all. She described a number of challenging experiences she had faced. Some customers would fall in love with her and become possessive of her. She had also experienced two instances of violence while selling sex. In each case, the customer tried to engage in a sexual act he hadn't paid for and wouldn't stop after repeated requests. One of the men threatened to find her where she lived. She hit the alarm button in her room and quickly had the other ladies and the administrators around her. She opened the door and pushed him out naked, throwing his clothes after him. The next time he returned she kicked him when he tried to come in. In the other instance, she fought a man off, squeezing his throat and kicking him. She took these negative experiences in stride: "No job is always fun," she said. Despite these experiences, Anka was never afraid while working in her window room. She felt safe given that the administrators were nearby and sounding her alarm would bring help right away. This was very different from selling sex in her home, where she would not have help if needed.

Anka understood that some women are forced into selling sex or forced to sell sex without condoms, but she explained that this is not the only story to be told about selling sex. She believed there was also another side—like her experience. She emphasized that "there are rotten apples everywhere," explaining that some women are abused in marriage, but this does not result in marriage being abolished. Along the same lines, the fact that some women are abused when selling sex, for her, was no grounds to make the practice illegal.

Spirituality and Morality

Anka reported that spirituality was important to her. She believed in mother nature. Selling sex did not conflict with her moral framework. In fact, Anka believed selling sex has a social function that benefits society. She described her diverse clientele: handicapped men, men traveling for work, men in sexless marriages, and those who only wanted to cuddle or sit together naked and have a conversation. She believed she provided a service to all of these customers. She even believed her function helps marriages. Her rationale was that if men are able to buy anal sex or something else their wives don't like, this prevents arguments at home.

Anka also described a darker side: men who brought their granddaughters clothing for her to wear, and want her to call them "grandpa." This would make her feel lousy, but she did it because she'd rather it be her than the granddaughters. She believed she was protecting these girls. Similarly, she believed customers who like sadomasochism are able to fulfill their fantasies by buying sex rather than by raping women in order to dominate them. In this sense, she was convinced her work prevents a variety of forms of abuse and violence. These are the reasons she believed selling sex should be legal, in addition to the more mundane argument that people are drawn to sex and that it shouldn't be taboo in society. If selling sex happens legally, she proposed, then the customer goes home satisfied and the woman gets to earn money—Anka saw no problem here.

Case 2: Jasmijn

At the time of the interview, Jasmijn was 24 years old, single, and did not have children. She had a high school education and had sold sex for 5 years in a number of settings, including in clubs, as an escort, and at her home. She earned all her income by selling sex, averaging about 1,000 euros a week on the basis of approximately 10 customers.

Motivation to Sell Sex

Jasmijn started selling sex because she felt it fit her personality. She had a high sex drive, a swinger mentality involving an open, non-monogamous attitude toward sex, and enjoyed having new experiences and getting to know new people. She continued selling sex because she enjoyed the variety she experienced in her work and also made good money. She had little desire to stop selling sex, but realized if she ever wanted a different job one day, this would be difficult given that she would not have a resume to show.

Consequences of Selling Sex

Jasmijn explained in detail the benefits she experienced from selling sex. After work she would feel full of self-confidence, calmer, more stable, and happier. She attributed developing social skills to selling sex, explaining how she used to be shy, but that selling sex encouraged her to become more open in her relationships with friends and in her interactions with strangers. She also reported becoming more involved in activities and starting to take better care of herself after starting to sell sex. She developed a healthier lifestyle by eating healthier and starting to exercise for the first time in her life. Her goal was to improve her appearance, but these actions additionally improved her attitude, all of which generated more customers for her. This description is consistent with some qualitative research indicating that middle-class women who sell sex indoors often describe a variety of advantages in their work, including that it encourages a sense of positive self-image and body image, greater comfort with one's sexuality, greater self-confidence, and the development of professional skills (Comte, 2014).

However, Jasmijn had also experienced some negative consequences of selling sex. At one time she worked in a sex club (brothel), which was not a good fit for her due to the high level of alcohol consumption associated with working in this setting. Her general practitioner helped her transition out of that setting into escort work.

The only other disadvantages she identified associated with selling sex were interpersonal and social in nature. First, she experienced negative effects in her romantic relationships, particularly when forming new relationships and disclosing her work. Some men would take advantage of this, with the idea that they could "get it for free." At other times, her choice to sell sex would result in her romantic relationships ending prematurely. Despite this, Jasmijn said she did not feel she lacked anything in her life. For the time being, she described herself as young and not ready to settle down.

In addition, Jasmijn described the prejudices she felt from society. Jasmijn had made the choice to speak very openly in her life about the fact that she sold sex. She liked sharing her work experiences and perspectives in an attempt to broaden people's understanding of the topic. She would regularly speak about this with friends, acquaintances, doctors, and other interested individuals.

Agency: Victims or willing workers?

Jasmijn reported actively choosing to sell sex for herself. She indicated that she truly enjoyed the work and did not see any problems with selling sex. Jasmijn described that every job has positive and negative sides and that each person has to evaluate how a job fits into his or her life (see section "A Rational Choice" of this chapter). When Jasmijn examined the impact of selling sex on her life, spirit, and emotions, she believed selling sex was the perfect job for her. What she liked about her choice was that she had the freedom to create change when she found herself in a rut. She could change brothels, start escorting, work with a webcam, or even organize events. She also explained that she could broaden her work and make it more fun by studying books on Tantra or Kama Sutra or learning from others.

Jasmijn indicated she desired to continue selling sex for many more years. Yet, similar to Anka, Jasmijn experienced mixed feelings to some extent. She described that the prejudices she felt from society sometimes made her doubt her choice to sell sex.

Empowerment Versus Exploitation

Jasmijn had experienced violence while selling sex, but continued to defend her desire to engage in this line of work. She indicated sex was the smallest part of the job for her; what she was really drawn to was the social aspects of the work and what she learned about human nature. For example, she would learn how different attitudes on her part would elicit different responses in customers. She also liked to observe how her own perspective would change on the basis of situations related to her customers. For example, she would notice that if she didn't have a lot of demand from customers, she would start to doubt herself and reevaluate her self-image. She valued gaining such insights. This reflects research findings that some women find selling sex meaningful and a path to personal growth (Bernstein, 2007).

Further, Jasmijn indicated selling sex gave her a lot of logistical flexibility she didn't have before. For example, she had suffered from insomnia for a long time, which had caused difficulties for schooling and jobs that required regular work hours. She explained selling sex solved this problem for her because she could create her own schedule. She indicated that she now had time to pursue education on the side. She said she couldn't even imagine working a 5–9 job and that it would be depressing to have to work for someone else.

Spirituality and Morality

Jasmijn explained that spirituality was somewhat important to her. She practiced Buddhism, and indicated that there was no conflict between her religious beliefs and her choice to sell sex. She also took an interest in the psychology of self-actualization, and believed selling sex helped her pursue her best self.

Discussion

The motivational factors described in these two case examples best represent personal interest and a rational choice. Commonalities we see in the stories of these two women are that they both chose to sell sex and viewed this as a positive choice in their lives. Both women also compared selling sex to other forms of work and argued that selling sex is a job like any other. Both described selling sex as having positive and negative sides. And, although both women argued for selling sex, both expressed some level of mixed feelings and ambivalence about their choice.

Another relevant theme is that both women spoke extensively about the social stigma surrounding selling sex (see Chap. 3). Each woman had to learn how to navigate having a job that other people don't understand. Each had chosen to respond to social stigma in very different ways. While Jasmijn chose to speak openly about selling sex and tried to educate others about it, Anka chose to keep her involvement in selling sex a secret as much as possible. Despite their differences, both women indicated what they appreciated most from others was an attitude of curiosity or interest rather than prejudice.

Researchers have pointed out that self-reports about selling sex are not bias-free (e.g., Vanwesenbeeck, 2001; Weatherall and Priestley, 2001), nevertheless, we see value in listening to the voices of women who sell sex and gaining insight into their perceptions of the themes discussed in this book. Of course, hearing from these two women cannot be generalized to others. What becomes clear from reviewing research on selling sex is that the environment in which the sale of sex takes place is very important to understanding a woman's experience (e.g., Rössler et al., 2010). In this case, the two interviewees sold sex legally in relatively safe conditions. This does not represent the majority of women who sell sex. Regardless, their stories are legitimate in their own right. What seemed important to these women was precisely the idea that not all instances of selling sex are the same. Anka used the Dutch expression: "*Je kan ons niet allemaal over één kam scheren,*" meaning that it's inappropriate to apply a broad-brush approach to the topic of selling sex. This sentiment is consistent with what researchers studying diverse groups of women who sell sex have found (Shaver, 2005).

In sum, the research indicates that in some settings, a noteworthy proportion of women report satisfaction with selling sex and describe deriving value from selling sex. Although this likely does not translate to women in all, or even most, locations and settings, the indication is that experiences with selling sex are not uniformly negative, and selling sex can be experienced as positive.

A Rational Choice

Not all women view sex the same way. Women who desire to reserve sex for intimate relationships are not likely to consider selling sex a desirable form of work for themselves. For women who are open to being paid for sex, the decision to start selling sex may be made in the same way as deciding to do any kind of work. Those who view selling sex as legitimate work argue that the choice to sell sex occurs through a rational process involving considering the advantages and disadvantages of selling sex against other work opportunities available (Esselstyn, 1968; Jeffrey & MacDonald, 2006; Rosen & Venkatesh, 2008; Sinha, 2015). This includes consideration of the previous themes of financial factors and personal enjoyment and other considerations in the cost-benefit analysis of selling sex compared to other work.

The most likely alternative, legal work choices for most women tend to be minimum-wage work in the service sector, such as waitressing, elder care, cleaning, call-center work, or work in the fast food industry (Jeffrey & MacDonald, 2006; Rosen & Venkatesh, 2008). Disadvantages of minimum wage work include low pay, a lack of independence, and high workplace discipline and control; service work may involve emotional burdens of working with difficult people and physical burdens of becoming tired or experiencing pain (e.g., Ehrenreich, 2001; Shipler, 2004). Some have also highlighted that workers can face sexual harassment in conventional work (Sinha, 2015). Selling sex shares some of these disadvantages in common with minimum wage work, including the possibility of low, unpredictable, or variable pay and physical burdens. Additional disadvantages identified by women who sell sex across a variety of countries (Australia, the Canadian Maritimes, the United States, and India) are that it is illegal in some jurisdictions,[3] including efforts to avoid police and

[2]Shaver (1994, 2005) has pointed out that distancing strategies are not unique to sex work, rather, professional distancing is often required as a form of emotional protection for many jobs, particularly in the caring professions.

[3]The legality of selling sex varies both between countries as well as within countries. For example, selling sex is illegal in all of the United States with the exception of certain rural counties in the state of Nevada. Selling sex is legal in much of Australia, though laws vary according to state and territory. Even in jurisdictions where selling sex may be legal or decriminalized, certain forms of

deal with potential legal consequences; it involves social stigma, including efforts to maintain separate identities in work and personal life; and it can involve safety concerns, including the risk of violence and the risk of contracting a sexually transmitted infection (STI; Bilardi et al., 2011; Jeffrey & MacDonald, 2006; Rosen & Venkatesh, 2008; Sinha, 2015).

With regard to the comparative advantages of selling sex over conventional work, similar themes have been highlighted in research from a variety of different countries (Australia, the US, the Canadian Maritimes, and India), including that selling sex offers more independence, the opportunity to be self-employed, the flexibility to set one's hours, the ability to avoid the structural constraints of conventional work, such as authority and discipline, and the ability to make more money in less time (Bilardi et al., 2011; Jeffrey & MacDonald, 2006; Rosen & Venkatesh, 2008; Sinha, 2015). Several of these studies have pointed out that the flexible working hours and comparatively greater pay for fewer hours worked allows for other commitments and obligations, such as caring for children or aging parents.

On this topic, we would be remiss not to note the controversy that exists regarding selling sex as a rational choice. Some maintain that the choice to sell sex is an artificial one. For example, Raymond (2013, p. 21) argued that "the response to the choice debate is *not* to deny that women are capable of choosing within contexts of powerlessness, but to question how much real value, worth, and power these so-called choices confer." A more moderate approach is offered by Rosen and Venkatesh (2008), who have illustrated that selling sex becomes a rational choice in low-wage economies with limited work opportunities. In the inner-city, selling sex offers "just enough money and flexibility to make the job worthwhile, and just enough autonomy and professional satisfaction to make it more attractive than other options" (Rosen & Venkatesh, 2008, p. 418). Yet, they note that being better than alternative options does not necessarily make selling sex itself an ideal or even a good choice, it's merely one that provides a basic level of satisfaction of needs. Further on the continuum are descriptions of women who sell sex even though they are educated, do not suffer from economic deprivation, and may even give up other work opportunities in order to sell sex (e.g., Bernstein 2007; Krumrei-Mancuso, 2017; Sanders, 2005; Sanders, Connelly, & King, 2016; see also the case examples provided in Text Box 2.1). Such accounts support the notion of a cost-benefit analysis that can lead some women to consider selling sex the more rational choice when compared to other legitimate alternatives.

Clinical Motivations

A counter perspective to the idea that selling sex is motivated by a rational choice, is the idea that selling sex is motivated by underlying clinical conditions. Clinical

---

commercial sex, such as street-based work, may be illegal. The legality of selling sex is discussed in more detail in Chap. 3.

perspectives about the psychological motivations for selling sex are often based on case examples of psychotherapy clients and support for these theories is difficult to establish empirically. Therefore, clinical theories may be relevant to individual women, but we strongly caution readers from concluding that a given clinical motivation is truly a theme among women who sell sex. Further, some of these theories clearly reflect a gender bias. We do not present these theories to advocate for their validity within the larger population of women selling sex. Rather, we simply seek to illustrate how some psychotherapists have sought to understand why their therapy clients began selling sex. In Chap. 7, we provide specific recommendations and tools for therapists and other helping professionals who work with women who sell sex, or have it in the past.

A number of theories have been developed in response to clinical work and research on the topic of childhood maltreatment (see Research in Depth on childhood maltreatment as a potential precursor to selling sex, in this chapter). One idea is that a history of sexual abuse makes it more likely that women will sell sex because they have learned to separate their emotions from sexual activity, making it easier for them to have sex for money. Another theory suggests that some women start selling sex to empower themselves in response to childhood abuse or adult sexual violence (Campbell, Ahrens, Sefl, & Clark, 2003; Nixon, Tutty, Downe, Gorkoff, & Ursel, 2002) or as a way to seek revenge and gratify aggressive impulses in response to victimization as a child (Hutto & Faulk, 2000; Kenny & Lane, 1996).

Another theme among clinical theories is that selling sex is motivated by women's relational needs. For example, some have suggested that women may associate love with sex and therefore sell sex as a way to feel valued (Nixon et al., 2002). Some theorists believe this motivation may be strongest for women who feel devalued in their daily life relationships (Campbell et al., 2003). Others have proposed that women may sell sex because they have difficulty maintaining emotional connections in personal relationships, and therefore seek an outlet for connectedness through body contact of a non-personal form (Hollender, 1961).

Finally, theories grounded within psychoanalytic frameworks draw on sexual or destructive motivations for selling sex. For example, some have suggested that selling sex is used to seek vicarious gratification of passive sexual wishes (e.g., Hutto & Faulk, 2000) or as a way to engage in self-destruction (Hollender, 1961). Selling sex as an expression of self-debasement is consistent with some self-reports of women who described selling sex to devalue themselves in response to being raped (Campbell et al., 2003).

Research in Depth: Childhood Maltreatment as a Potential Precursor to Selling Sex

In addition to the mostly acute motivational factors we have described thus far, we will also consider a more distal factor that has been examined as a potential precursor to selling sex. We will provide a more in-depth look at the complex, controversial, and frequently studied topic of childhood maltreatment in relation to selling sex. It is important to note that childhood maltreatment is only one of many youth variables that might function as a precursor to selling sex. For example, early sexual initiation, running away from home, juvenile arrests, skipping school, and getting in trouble at school have all been associated with subsequently selling sex (Wilson & Widom, 2010). We decided to highlight the topic of childhood maltreatment because it has been examined most extensively in the literature. Childhood physical and sexual abuse have both been studied extensively as precursors to women starting to sell sex, with the most focus on childhood sexual abuse. Childhood emotional abuse and neglect have also been examined to a lesser extent. Within this body of research, the cutoff age for childhood maltreatment is typically 16 years, however, some researchers examine abuse and neglect that occur until age 15 or 18.

Self-reports of Childhood Maltreatment as a Reason for Selling Sex

Around the 1980s there was a research emphasis on examining self-reported causal attributions of childhood abuse leading to selling sex. For example, in a study of women formerly selling sex on the street, over half of the sample indicated that childhood sexual abuse had heavily influenced their decision to start selling sex (Bagley & Young, 1987). In studies in which youth are included within the sample, this rate is often even higher. For example, among a sample of which the majority were youth who used to sell sex on the street,[4] 70% indicated that sexual abuse had affected their decision to start selling sex (Silbert & Pines, 1983). Although it is important to understand the reasons to which women attribute starting to sell sex, relying strictly on self-reported causal attributions about childhood maltreatment can be problematic, given that this assumes women are able to accurately infer such causal links from early life events.

Comparisons to Women in the General Population

To explore the link between childhood maltreatment and selling sex, some studies have aimed to establish whether rates of childhood maltreatment are higher among women who sell sex than among those who don't. A number of studies comparing women who have sold sex with women in the general population have concluded that those who sell sex have experienced more childhood maltreatment. For example, a

[4]The ages of the sample ranged from 10 to 46, with an average age of 22 years. The majority of participants in this study were youths.

Canadian study found much higher rates of physical, sexual, and emotional abuse, and neglect during childhood among those who had sold sex compared to a random sample of individuals from the same area (Bagley & Young, 1987). The results also indicated that women who had sold sex were significantly more likely to have experienced more types of abuse than those who had not sold sex. Similarly, a study from New Zealand comparing women who had sold sex to women in a random community survey indicated that those who had sold sex were more likely to have been raped before the age of 16 (Potter et al., 1999).[5]

If we examine the prevalence rates of childhood abuse among women who sell sex from research from around the world, we see that the rates vary widely across studies. Physical abuse is reported by proportions of samples of women who sell sex around 24% on the low end (Clarke, Clarke, Roe-Sepowitz, & Fey, 2012) and 55% on the high end (Roe-Sepowitz, 2012). This number tends to be higher among samples that include minors (e.g., 72% reported by Farley, Lynne, & Cotton, 2005).[6] These rates compare to 22% of females in the general population who report childhood physical abuse according to a large meta-analysis[7] of self-report research from around the world (Stoltenborgh, Bakermans-Kranenburg, van IJzendoorn, & Alink, 2013).

Sexual abuse is reported by proportions of samples of women who sell sex around 25% on the low end (Sanders, 2001) and 79% on the high end (Roe-Sepowitz, 2012). This compares to 18% of females in the general population who report childhood sexual abuse according to a large meta-analysis of self-report research from around the world (Stoltenborgh, van IJzendoorn, Euser, & Bakermans-Kranenburg, 2011).

Finally, emotional abuse is reported by proportions of samples of women who sell sex around 35% on the low end (Clarke et al., 2012) and 62% on the high end (Surratt et al., 2004). This compares to 38% of females in the general population who report childhood emotional abuse according to a large meta-analysis self-report research from around the world (Stoltenborgh, Bakermans-Kranenburg, Alink, & Van Ijzendoorn, 2012).

These comparisons make clear that some samples of women who sell sex have experienced childhood abuse at much higher rates than women in the general population, whereas other samples of women who sell sex are roughly equivalent to women in the general population with regard to their rate of exposure to childhood abuse. The vastly different rates of abuse across samples of women who sell sex highlights the heterogeneity among these women.

The overall conclusions that can be drawn from this type of research is limited by the fact that random samples from the general population are often not ideal comparison groups for women who sell sex. Some of the research responses to this problem have been to employ more specific comparison samples, use prospective cohort designs, and examine age of entry into selling sex. Next, we will consider findings from each of these methodologies.

---

[5]The sample of women who sold sex started at age 16, with an average age of 29 years.

[6]The mean age of this sample was 28 years, but participants as young as 13 years were included.

[7]Meta-analysis is a widely-used research synthesis method that permits results from multiple primary studies to be statistically combined.

Studies with Specific Comparison Samples

Given that there may be important differences between women who sell sex and samples of women from the general population, a number of studies have attempted to compare rates of childhood maltreatment between those who do and do not sell sex within samples that share similar life experiences and circumstances. Such methods have been more likely to show no significant differences or mixed results with regard to whether childhood maltreatment is associated with a greater likelihood of selling sex. This research has primarily targeted women facing challenges of various kinds, including poverty, criminal involvement, sexually transmitted infections, and substance abuse. Next, we will summarize some of the key findings from these literatures.

Recruitment in Poor, Urban Settings

A study of poor women recruited on the street near public housing and drug and sex exchange sites, indicated that those with and without a history of childhood sexual abuse did not differ with regard to whether they had sold sex within the past 30 days (Mosack, Randolph, Dickson-Gomez, Abbott, Smith & Weeks, 2010). Similar results have been found among matched samples of youths who were recruited from the same neighborhoods, outreach programs, residential treatment centers, and detention facilities. Both samples experienced high rates of childhood sexual abuse, and female youth (mean age of 16.3) who had received money for sex did not differ significantly from the youth (mean age of 15.7) who had not received money for sex with regard to the incidence, frequency, or duration of childhood sexual abuse, nor were there significant differences in the average age of onset of victimization, the nature of the perpetrator, and whether force was used (Nadon, Koverola, & Schludermann, 1998). Furthermore, in this study, those who had neveer received money for sex reported significantly higher rates of childhood physical abuse than those who had received money for sex (71 vs. 45%). Those who had never received money for sex also reported a greater number of physical violence acts.

Offender Samples

Among women in trouble with the law, some, but not all, studies have indicated links between childhood maltreatment and selling sex. In a large United States study of female criminal offenders, those who had ever sold sex were more likely to have witnessed violence growing up and were more likely to have been a victim of domestic violence and sexual assault as children, even when controlling participants' age, race, education, partner status, employment, and income (Perdue et al., 2012). Likewise, in another large study of female jail detainees (mostly adults, but starting at age 17 years), childhood sexual abuse came close to doubling the odds of selling sex (McClanahan, McClelland, Abram, & Teplin, 1999). That is, 44% of detainees who had experienced childhood sexual abuse had sold sex, compared to 28% of detainees with no history of sexual abuse. In contrast, another study of female criminal offenders indicated a host of childhood factors were not related to whether a woman had sold or traded sex. These included physical, psychological, or sexual abuse or neglect by caregivers, nonfamilial physical or sexual violence, and witnessing violence inside or outside of the home (DeHart et al., 2014).

STI Samples

Results are also mixed among women with STIs. For example, among women at an STI clinic, prepubertal rape was more commonly reported by women who sold sex (32%) than by those who did not (13%), even though both groups were demographically similar (Potterat, Rothenberg, Muth, Darrow, & Phillips-Plummer, 1998). On the other hand, a smaller study of two groups of women with gonorrhea who were matched for age, race, and sexual practices indicated that the number of those who had experienced physical abuse and sexual abuse as children was almost identical between those who had and had not sold sex (Potterat Phillips, Rothenberg, & Darrow, 1985). In fact, the percentage of women who had experienced sexual abuse as children and the percentage of those who had been raped prior to first intercourse was greater among those who had not sold sex than among those who had.

Substance Abuse Samples

Among substance abusing women, the results are, again, mixed. In American studies of substance abusing women, significant links have been observed between childhood sexual abuse and trading sex for money or drugs (e.g., El-Bassel, Simoni, Cooper, Gilbert, & Schilling, 2001; Vaddiparti et al., 2006). In a study of heavy drinking and drug using women, those who had ever traded sex for money, drugs, food, clothes, or housing were more likely to report sexual abuse occurring prior to age 15 (Vaddiparti et al., 2006). Although both those who had and had not traded sex reported high rates of childhood sexual abuse, all assessed forms of abuse were reported significantly more often by those who had traded sex compared to those who had not, including being forced to kiss or touch someone in a sexual way (35 vs. 22%), being kissed or touched in a sexual way against their will (42 vs. 31%), and being raped (30 vs. 21%).

Other studies have not observed significant links. Among a sample of drug using women in Scotland, those who had and had not sold sex did not differ with regard to whether they had experienced emotional, physical, or sexual abuse in childhood (Gilchrist, Gruer, & Atkinson, 2005). Similarly, a longitudinal study from the United States of individuals receiving outpatient substance abuse treatment found that neither a history of sexual nor physical abuse was predictive of selling sex (Fiorentine, Pilati, & Hillhouse, 1999). Finally, some studies finding higher rates of sexual abuse among those who had sold sex compared to those who had not, did not find differences for childhood physical abuse (operationalized as abuse from a parent or guardian requiring medical attention; Vaddiparti et al., 2006).

Making Sense of the Research Using Specific Comparison Samples

The majority of research employing specific comparison samples has observed higher rates of childhood maltreatment among women who have sold sex compared to those who have not sold sex, but the findings are far from unanimous. A potential explanatory variable in the link between childhood abuse and selling sex is post-traumatic stress disorder (PTSD). For example, a large study of African American women who used crack cocaine initially indicated histories of childhood physical and sexual abuse were both associated with trading sex for money or drugs in adulthood (Edwards, Halpern, & Wechsberg, 2006). Even when controlling age, marital status, the number of friends who used drugs, homelessness, and unemployment, women who were abused in childhood were more likely to trade sex than women who did not experience childhood abuse. However, when PTSD was added to the analyses together with all other variables, childhood abuse was no longer a significant predictor of trading sex for money or drugs. Thus, it seems that having experienced childhood abuse may be only an indirect indicator of a greater likelihood of selling sex, and what matters more in predicting selling sex is whether or not a woman experiences PTSD following the abuse.

A limitation of the body of literature employing similar comparison samples is that studies have primarily examined women with particular life challenges, including poverty, incarceration, STIs, and substance abuse. Therefore, this work sheds light on links between childhood maltreatment and selling sex only for women involved in high-risk situations or behaviors and leaves open the question as to whether there are links between childhood sexual abuse and selling sex for women who are not facing similar difficulties. An alternative research methodology that is not limited in this sense involves employing a prospective design, which we will consider next.

Prospective Cohort Design

A response to the concern about employing inequivalent comparison groups is to make use of matching techniques. Widom and Kuhns (1996) conducted a prospective cohorts study in which they followed into adulthood a sample of physically and sexually abused and neglected children who were matched to a control group of children who had not been maltreated on the basis of sex, age, race, and social class. This approach is rare because of the length of time it takes to conduct the research and be able to draw conclusions. However, this research design is able to provide more trustworthy results because it minimizes some of the confounding factors that otherwise make it difficult to draw conclusions. The results indicated that childhood abuse and neglect were significant predictors of selling sex for women. After controlling age, race, gender, and socioeconomic status, childhood sexual abuse and neglect were predictive of selling sex, but childhood physical abuse only approached significance. This research design is explored in more depth in Text Box 2.2.

Text Box 2.2 Research Note: Examining Childhood Maltreatment as a Precursor to Selling Sex with a Prospective Cohort Study of Boys and Girls

Difficulty establishing causality between childhood sexual abuse and selling sex results from the inability to randomly assign participants to groups. To simulate this as closely as possible, Wilson and Widom (2010) conducted analyses based on a large prospective cohort design in which abused and neglected boys and girls were matched on the basis of age, sex, race/ethnicity and family social class with a control group of non-abused, non-neglected boys and girls (ages 0–11). Both groups were followed into adulthood (average age of 29 years), the assumption being that the two groups would be similar to one another outside of the experience of abuse or neglect. This design allows links between childhood maltreatment and selling sex to be examined without the interference of a number of potentially confounding variables.

Path model analyses indicated that those with documented cases of childhood physical or sexual abuse or neglect were more than twice as likely than the control participants to start selling sex by young adulthood. The strongest links were observed for childhood physical abuse and neglect in predicting selling sex. This particular publication must be interpreted with some caution for the purpose of the current chapter due to the fact that approximately half of the sample consisted of males and the genders were not analyzed separately. However, another article on the same data confirmed that childhood abuse and neglect were predictive of selling sex in early adulthood for women and, in fact, not for men (Widom & Kuhns, 1996).

Interestingly, four youth characteristics partially accounted for the relationship between childhood abuse and subsequently selling sex: early sexual initiation, running away, juvenile crime, and school problems. However, when all these youth behaviors were entered together into a model, only the path from early sexual initiation remained significant in predicting selling sex. Thus, of all the variables assessed, becoming sexually active before the age of 15 was the single strongest predictor of later starting to sell sex among those who had experienced childhood physical or sexual abuse or neglect.

This prospective cohort study highlights three important messages. First, children who experience physical or sexual abuse or neglect are much more likely than children who are not maltreated to sell sex by young adulthood. Second, although quite a bit of research has emphasized sexual abuse as a risk factor for selling sex, this study found childhood physical abuse and neglect to be stronger predictors of selling sex than sexual abuse. Finally, it seems that sexual relationships in early adolescence are a relevant factor associated with selling sex among those who were maltreated as children.

Age of Entry

A final antidote to the pitfall of incommensurable comparison groups is to conduct research without a comparison group, assessing strictly women who have sold sex, to explore whether childhood maltreatment relates to the age at which women start selling sex. For example, in a United States study of women who had sold sex on the street, childhood emotional abuse was associated with starting to sell sex at a younger age (Roe-Sepowitz, 2012). Similar research has indicated that childhood risk factors tend to go together and that their effects are equivalent to one another with regard to starting to sell sex. For example, among a sample of women who had sold sex on the street in Phoenix, childhood sexual abuse, childhood physical abuse, and childhood parental drug or alcohol abuse were all highly correlated, and equally strong in predicting the age at which the women started selling sex (Kramer & Berg, 2003). Experiencing any of these risk factors in comparison to none of these risk factors was associated with selling sex at a younger age.

Reasons for Mixed Findings Regarding Childhood Maltreatment and Selling Sex

In reflecting on this body of literature as a whole, it is clear that the statistics vary, sometimes suggesting that women who sell sex do, and other times suggesting they do not, experience more childhood maltreatment than women who do not sell sex. The inconsistencies in the findings may relate to a number of factors, including differing conceptual and operational definitions of abuse and uncontrolled mediating variables.

To illustrate the relevance of the way in which abuse is defined and measured, a study found that there were no significant differences between a sample of women who sold sex and a random community sample with regard to the experience of childhood genital fondling but there were significant differences with regard to penetrative childhood sexual abuse, with 32% of the women who sold sex having experienced attempted rape before the age of 16 (with 25% of the sample experiencing complete penetration), compared to 9% of the community sample of women who had experienced attempted rape before the age of 16 (with 5% of this sample experiencing complete penetration; Potter et al., 1999). Thus, different findings emerge depending on the way childhood maltreatment is defined and assessed. Moreover, even when *rates* of abuse do not differ between women who have and have not experienced childhood maltreatment, the specific details of abuse may be different. Research has indicated that sexual abuse that is more frequent, lasts a longer period of time, begins at a younger age, occurs by multiple offenders, has sadistic or masochistic qualities, or results in a negative reaction within the victim is more likely to be associated with selling sex (Bagley & Young, 1987).

Unfortunately, even the best available research designs are not able to determine with certainty whether childhood maltreatment exists in a causal sequence with selling sex. Even if causality is suggested, it may occur through other variables. For example, research has begun to examine how childhood maltreatment may be linked to selling sex via family characteristics, running away from home, skipping school, using drugs, or getting in trouble with the law (see Text Box 2.2). Other potential mediating variables include the psychosocial impact of abuse in the woman's life. Research has shown that traumatic childhood abuse is associated with lower psychosocial functioning and quality of life (Wu, Schairer, Dello, & Grella, 2010) and more serious mental illness (Surratt, Kurtz, Chen, & Mooss, 2012). Among women who sell sex, having experienced childhood abuse or neglect is associated with more mental health symptoms in adulthood, such as depression and PTSD (Choi, Klein, Shin, & Lee, 2009; Gilchrist et al., 2005; Sanders, 2004; Ulibarri et al., 2009). Thus, links between childhood maltreatment and selling sex may result from conditions such as PTSD, depression, or anxiety, that develop in response to maltreatment and become antecedents to selling sex. This paints the picture of a web of interrelated factors. For example, childhood maltreatment may result in any number of difficulties, including lower self-esteem or self-efficacy; feelings of worthlessness, hopelessness, helplessness, inferiority, or internalized shame; difficulty processing emotions; lack of healthy coping skills; social alienation; and real or imagined social stigma. All of these factors may impact selling sex directly or via other factors such as academic success and work opportunities. In addition, childhood abuse has a connection to substance use (Wu et al., 2010), which relates to another motivation for selling sex already discussed. To date, little research has directly evaluated these psychological factors that relate to how and why childhood sexual abuse may be associated with selling sex. An exception comes from Mosack and colleagues (2010) who examined how a woman's sense of control relates to selling sex. They found among women with a history of childhood sexual abuse, that those who had less control in their relationships with their significant others and a more external locus of control for acquiring an STI, were more likely to sell sex. In contrast, relationship control and locus of control for STI were not related to selling sex among women without a history of childhood sexual abuse. Many of the mental health variables noted here as potential mediators between childhood maltreatment and selling sex are explored in more depth in Chap. 4.

Discussion

The research literature about why women sell sex includes a broad range of motivational factors that encompass themes of powerlessness and passivity, as well as agency and control. Some studies emphasize external influences, such as poverty, family obligations, and limited alternatives, whereas other studies emphasize rational choice and personal interest leading to selling sex. An important insight gained by reviewing the reasons women sell sex is the great diversity that exists among women. The various reasons for starting to sell may differ between studies on the basis of context, location, and culture. Moreover, there is diversity not only across studies, but also within studies on the basis of individual participants' life experiences and personal values. Taken one level further, there are multiple, sometimes conflicting experiences within individual women, as well. This is evidenced within qualitative research, when women within the same interview might in one moment describe themselves as autonomous agents who are in control of their choice to sell sex, and in another moment use the language of being passive and powerless objects for sale (e.g., Weatherall & Priestley, 2001). This highlights that women's experiences are often multifaceted. For example, women may start selling sex to work for themselves in a setting where they set the rules, yet they may also experience coercion and exploitation at times. Or, a woman may begin selling sex for one reason, yet continue selling sex for another. Understanding the diversity of factors that influence women to start selling sex involves understanding not only the varied experiences that exist across populations, but also the disparate factors that influence any given woman to start selling sex.

References

Abramovich, E. (2005). Childhood sexual abuse as a risk factor for subsequent involvement in sex work: A review of empirical findings. *Journal of Psychology & Human Sexuality, 17,* 131–146. https://doi.org/10.1300/J056v17n01_08.

Ariyabuddhiphongs, V., & Li, J. (2012). Sacrifice and optimism among Thai masseuses: The mediating role of pride. *International Perspectives in Psychology: Research, Practice, Consultation, 1,* 154–164. https://doi.org/10.1037/a0029233.

Bagley, C., & Young, L. (1987). Juvenile prostitution and child sexual abuse: A controlled study. *Canadian Journal of Community Mental Health, 6,* 5–26. https://doi.org/10.7870/cjcmh-1987-0001.

Bernstein, E. (2007). Sex work for the middle classes. *Sexualities, 10,* 473–488. https://doi.org/10.1177/1363460707080984.

Bilardi, J. E., Miller, A., Hocking, J. S., Keogh, L., Cummings, R., Chen, M. Y., et al. (2011). The job satisfaction of female sex workers working in licensed brothels in Victoria, Australia. *Journal of Sexual Medicine, 8,* 116–122. https://doi.org/10.1111/j.1743-6109.2010.01967.x.

Bovenkerk, F., & Van San, M. (2011). Loverboys in the Amsterdam red light district: A realist approach to the study of a moral panic. *Crime, Media, Culture, 7,* 185–199. https://doi.org/10.1177/1741659011412124.

Campbell, R., Ahrens, C. E., Sefl, T., & Clark, M. L. (2003). The relationship between adult sexual assault and prostitution: An exploratory analysis. *Violence and Victims, 18,* 299–317. https://doi.org/10.1891/vivi.2003.18.3.299.

Choi, H., Klein, C., Shin, M., & Lee, H. (2009). Posttraumatic stress disorder (PTSD) and disorders of extreme stress (DESNOS) symptoms following prostitution and childhood abuse. *Violence Against Women, 15,* 933–951. https://doi.org/10.1177/1077801209335493.

Clarke, R. J., Clarke, E. A., Roe-Sepowitz, D., & Fey, R. (2012). Age at entry into prostitution: Relationship to drug use, race, suicide, education level, childhood abuse, and family experiences. *Journal of Human Behavior in the Social Environment, 22,* 270–289. https://doi.org/10.1080/10911359.2012.655583.

Cobbina, J. E., & Oselin, S. S. (2011). It's not only for the money: An analysis of adolescent versus adult entry into street prostitution. *Sociological Inquiry, 81,* 310–332. https://doi.org/10.1111/j.1475-682X.2011.00375.x.

Comte, J. (2014). Decriminalization of sex work: Feminist discourses. *Sexuality and Culture, 18,* 196–217. https://doi.org/10.1007/s12119-013-9174-5.

DeHart, D., Lynch, S., Belknap, J., Dass-Brailsford, P., & Green, B. (2014). Life history models of female offending: The roles of serious mental illness and trauma in women's pathways to jail. *Psychology of Women Quarterly, 38,* 138–151. https://doi.org/10.1177/0361684313494357.

Edwards, J. M., Halpern, C. T., & Wechsberg, W. M. (2006). Correlates of exchanging sex for drugs or money among women who use crack cocaine. *AIDS Education and Prevention, 18,* 420–429. https://doi.org/10.1521/aeap.2006.18.5.420.

Ehrenreich, B. (2001). *Nickel and dimed: On (not) getting by in America.* New York: Henry Holt.

El-Bassel, N., Simoni, J. M., Cooper, D. K., Gilbert, L., & Schilling, R. F. (2001). Sex trading and psychological distress among women on methadone. *Psychology of Addictive Behaviors, 15,* 177–184. https://doi.org/10.1037//0893-164X.15.3.177.

Esselstyn, T. C. (1968). Prostitution in the United States. *Annals of the American Academy of Political and Social Science, 376,* 123–135. https://doi.org/10.1177/000271626837600112.

Farley, M. (2006). Prostitution, trafficking, and cultural amnesia: What we must *not know* in order to keep the business of sexual exploitation running smoothly. *Yale Journal of Law and Feminism, 18,* 109–144.

Farley, M., Lynne, J., & Cotton, A. J. (2005). Prostitution in Vancouver: Violence and the colonization of First Nations women. *Transcultural Psychiatry, 42,* 242–271. https://doi.org/10.1177/1363461505052667.

Farley, M., Cotton, A., Lynne, J., Zumbeck, S., Spiwak, F., Reyes, M. E., … Sezgin, U. (2003). Prostitution and trafficking in nine countries: An update on violence and posttraumatic stress disorder. *Journal of Trauma Practice, 2*(3/4), 33–74. https://doi.org/10.1300/j189v02n03_03.

Fiorentine, R., Pilati, M. L., & Hillhouse, M. P. (1999). Drug treatment outcomes: Investigating the long-term effects of sexual and physical abuse histories. *Journal of Psychoactive Drugs, 31,* 363–372. https://doi.org/10.1080/02791072.1999.10471766.

Gilchrist, G., Gruer, L., & Atkinson, J. (2005). Comparison of drug use and psychiatric morbidity between prostitute and non-prostitute female drug users in Glasgow, Scotland. *Addictive Behaviors, 30,* 1019–1023. https://doi.org/10.1016/j.addbeh.2004.09.003.

Goldenberg, S. M., Engstrom, D., Rolon, M. L., Silverman, J. G., & Strathdee, S. A. (2013). Sex workers perspectives on strategies to reduce sexual exploitation and HIV risk: A qualitative study in Tijuana, Mexico. *PLoS One, 8*(8). https://doi.org/10.1371/journal.pone.0072982.

Harding, R., & Hamilton, P. (2009). Working girls: Abuse or choice in street-level sex work? A study of homeless women in Nottingham. *British Journal of Social Work, 39,* 1118–1137. https://doi.org/10.1093/bjsw/bcm157.

Hollender, M. H. (1961). Prostitution, the body, and human relatedness. *The International Journal of Psychoanalysis, 42,* 404–413.

Hutto, B., & Faulk, R. (2000). Psychodynamics of a prostitute: A case report. *Bulletin of the Menninger Clinic, 64,* 409–423.

Jeffrey, L. A., & MacDonald, G. (2006). "It's the money, honey": The economy of sex work in the Maritimes. *Canadian Review of Sociology and Anthropology, 43,* 313–327. https://doi.org/10.1111/j.1755-618x.2006.tb02227.x.

Kenny, M. C., & Lane, R. C. (1996). Memoirs of a drug-abusing prostitute: Dynamics and treatment considerations in a case of intergenerational child abuse. *Journal of Contemporary Psychotherapy, 26,* 361–378. https://doi.org/10.1007/BF02312916.

Kramer, L. A., & Berg, E. C. (2003). A survival analysis of timing of entry into prostitution: The differential impact of race, educational level, and childhood/adolescent risk factors. *Sociological Inquiry, 73,* 511–528. https://doi.org/10.1111/1475-682X.00069.

Krumrei-Mancuso, E. J. (2017). Sex work and mental health: A study of women in the Netherlands. *Archives of Sexual Behavior, 46,* 1843–1856.

MacKinnon, C. A. (1993). Prostitution and civil rights. *Michigan Journal of Gender & Law, 1,* 13–31.

McCaghy, C. H., & Hou, C. (1994). Family affiliations and prostitution in a cultural context: Career onsets of Taiwanese prostitutes. *Archives of Sexual Behavior, 23,* 251–265. https://doi.org/10.1007/BF01541562.

McClanahan, S. F., McClelland, G. M., Abram, K. M., & Teplin, L. A. (1999). Pathways into prostitution among female jail detainees and their implications for mental health service. *Psychiatric Services, 50,* 1606–1613. https://doi.org/10.1176/ps.50.12.1606.

Morris, M. D., Lemus, H., Wagner, K. D., Martinez, G., Lozada, R., Gómez, R., et al. (2013). Factors associated with pathways toward concurrent sex work and injection drug use among female sex workers who inject drugs in northern Mexico. *Addiction, 108,* 161–170. https://doi.org/10.1111/j.1360-0443.2012.04016.x.

Mosack, K. E., Randolph, M. E., Dickson-Gomez, J., Abbott, M., Smith, E., & Weeks, M. R. (2010). Sexual risk-taking among high-risk urban women with and without histories of childhood sexual abuse: Mediating effects of contextual factors. *Journal of Child Sexual Abuse, 19,* 43–61. https://doi.org/10.1080/10538710903485591.

Murphy, L. (2010). Understanding the social and economic contexts surrounding women engaged in street-level prostitution. *Issues in Mental Health Nursing, 31,* 775–784. https://doi.org/10.3109/01612840.2010.524345.

Nadon, S. M., Koverola, C., & Schludermann, E. H. (1998). Antecedents to prostitution: Childhood victimization. *Journal of Interpersonal Violence, 13,* 206–221. https://doi.org/10.1177/088626098013002003.

Nixon, K., Tutty, L., Downe, P., Gorkoff, K., & Ursel, J. (2002). The everyday occurrence: Violence in the lives of girls exploited through prostitution. *Violence Against Women, 8,* 1016–1043. https://doi.org/10.1177/107780120200800902.

Oerton, S., & Phoenix, J. (2001). Sex/bodywork: Discourses and practices. *Sexualities, 4,* 387–412. https://doi.org/10.1177/136346001004004001.

Perdue, T. R., Williamson, C., Ventura, L. A., Hairston, T. R., Osborne, L. T., Laux, J. M., … Nathan, V. M. (2012). Offenders who are mothers with and without experience in prostitution: Differences in historical trauma, current stressors, and physical and mental health differences. *Women's Health Issues, 22,* e195–e200. https://doi.org/10.1016/j.whi.2011.08.010.

Platt, L., Grenfell, P., Bonell, C., Creighton, S., Wellings, K., … Rhodes, T. (2011). Risk of sexually transmitted infections and violence among indoor-working female sex workers in London: The effect of migration from Eastern Europe. *Sexually Transmitted Infections, 87,* 377–384. https://doi.org/10.1136/sti.2011.049544.

Potter, K., Martin, J., & Romans, S. (1999). Early developmental experiences of female sex workers: A comparative study. *Australian and New Zealand Journal of Psychiatry, 33,* 935–940. https://doi.org/10.1046/j.1440-1614.1999.00655.x.

Potterat, J. J., Phillips, L., Rothenberg, R. B., & Darrow, W. (1985). On becoming a prostitute: An exploratory case-comparison study. *Journal of Sex Research, 21,* 329–335. https://doi.org/10.1080/00224498509551271.

Potterat, J. J., Rothenberg, R. B., Muth, S. Q., Darrow, W. W., & Phillips-Plummer, L. (1998). Pathways to prostitution: The chronology of sexual and drug abuse milestones. *Journal of Sex Research, 35,* 333–340. https://doi.org/10.1080/00224499809551951.

Rael, C. T. (2015). Perceptions of sex work-related stigma in female sex workers from the Dominican Republic: Implications for HIV interventions. *Sexuality and Culture, 19,* 674–684. https://doi.org/10.1007/s12119-015-9284-3.

Raymond, J. G. (2013). *Not a choice, not a job: Exposing the myths about the prostitution trade.* Washington, DC: Potomac Books.

Roe-Sepowitz, D. E. (2012). Juvenile entry into prostitution: The role of emotional abuse. *Violence Against Women, 18,* 562–579. https://doi.org/10.1177/1077801212453140.

Rosen, E., & Venkatesh, S. A. (2008). A "perversion" of choice: Sex work offers *just enough* in Chicago's urban ghetto. *Journal of Contemporary Ethnography, 37,* 417–441. https://doi.org/10.1177/0891241607309879.

Rössler, W. W., Koch, U. U., Lauber, C. C., Hass, A. K., Altwegg, M. M., Ajdacic-Gross, V. V., et al. (2010). The mental health of female sex workers. *Acta Psychiatrica Scandinavica, 122,* 143–152. https://doi.org/10.1111/j.1600-0447.2009.01533.x.

Roxburgh, A., Degenhardt, L., & Copeland, J. (2006). Posttraumatic stress disorder among female street-based sex workers in the greater Sydney area, Australia. *BMC Psychiatry, 6,* 24. https://doi.org/10.1186/1471-244X-6-24.

Sanders, T. (2001). Female street workers, sexual violence, and protection strategies. *Journal of Sexual Aggression, 7,* 5–18. https://doi.org/10.1080/13552600108413318.

Sanders, T. (2002). VI. The condom as psychological barrier: Female sex workers and emotional management. *Feminism & Psychology, 12,* 561–566. https://doi.org/10.1177/0959353502012004016.

Sanders, T. (2004). A continuum of risk? The management of health, physical and emotional risks by female sex workers. *Sociology of Health & Illness, 26,* 557–574. https://doi.org/10.1111/j.0141-9889.2004.00405.x.

Sanders, T. (2005). "It's just acting": Sex workers' strategies for capitalizing on sexuality. *Gender, Work and Organization, 12,* 319–342. https://doi.org/10.1111/j.1468-0432.2005.00276.x.

Sanders, T., Connelly, L., & King, L. J. (2016). On our own terms: The working conditions of internet sex workers in the UK. *Sociological Research Online, 21*(4). https://doi.org/10.5153/sro.4152.

Seib, C., Dunne, M. P., Fischer, J., & Najman, J. M. (2012). Predicting the job satisfaction of female sex workers in Queensland, Australia. *International Journal of Sexual Health, 24,* 99–111.

Shaver, F. M. (1994). The regulation of prostitution: Avoiding the morality traps. *Canadian Journal of Law and Society, 9,* 123–145. https://doi.org/10.1017/s0829320100003537.

Shaver, F. M. (2005). Sex work research: Methodological and ethical challenges. *Journal of Interpersonal Violence, 20,* 296–319. https://doi.org/10.1177/0886260504274340.

Shipler, D. (2004). *The working poor: Invisible in America.* New York: Alfred Knopf.

Sinha, S. (2015). Reasons for women's entry into sex work: A case study of Kolkata, India. *Sexuality and Culture, 19,* 216–235. https://doi.org/10.1007/s12119-014-9256-z.

Stoltenborgh, M., van IJzendoorn, M. H., Euser, E. M., & Bakermans-Kranenburg, M. J. (2011). A global perspective on child sexual abuse: Meta-analysis of prevalence around the world. *Child Maltreatment, 16,* 79–101. https://doi.org/10.1177/1077559511403920.

Stoltenborgh, M., Bakermans-Kranenburg, M.J., Alink, L.A., & Van Ijzendoorn, M.H. (2012). The universality of childhood emotional abuse: A meta-analysis of worldwide prevalence. *Journal of Aggression, Maltreatment & Trauma, 21,* 870–890. https://doi.org/10.1080/10926771.2012.708014.

Stoltenborgh, M., Bakermans-Kranenburg, M. J., van IJzendoorn, M. H., & Alink, L. A. (2013). Cultural–geographical differences in the occurrence of child physical abuse? A meta-analysis of global prevalence. *International Journal of Psychology, 48,* 81–94. https://doi.org/10.1080/00207594.2012.697165.

Suresh, G., Furr, L., & Srikrishnan, A. (2009). An assessment of the mental health of street-based sex workers in Chennai, India. *Journal of Contemporary Criminal Justice, 25,* 186–201. https://doi.org/10.4135/9788132114109.n16.

Surratt, H. L., Inciardi, J. A., Kurtz, S. P., & Kiley, M. C. (2004). Sex work and drug use in a subculture of violence. *Crime & Delinquency, 50,* 43–59. https://doi.org/10.1177/0011128703258875.

Surratt, H. L., Kurtz, S. P., Chen, M., & Mooss, A. (2012). HIV risk among female sex workers in Miami: The impact of violent victimization and untreated mental illness. *AIDS Care, 24,* 553–561. https://doi.org/10.1080/09540121.2011.630342.

Thappa, D., Singh, N., & Kaimal, S. (2007). Prostitution in India and its role in the spread of HIV infection. *Indian Journal of Sexually Transmitted Diseases, 28,* 69–75. https://doi.org/10.4103/0253-7184.39007.

Ulibarri, M. D., Semple, S. J., Rao, S., Strathdee, S. A., Fraga-Vallejo, M. A., Bucardo, J., … Patterson, T. L. (2009). History of abuse and psychological distress symptoms among female sex workers in two Mexico–U.S. border cities. *Violence and Victims, 24,* 399–413. https://doi.org/10.1891/0886-6708.24.3.399.

Vaddiparti, K., Bogetto, J., Callahan, C., Abdallah, A. B., Spitznagel, E. L., & Cottler, L. B. (2006). The effects of childhood trauma on sex trading in substance using women. *Archives of Sexual Behavior, 35,* 451–459. https://doi.org/10.1007/s10508-006-9044-4.

Vanwesenbeeck, I. (2001). Another decade of social scientific work on sex work: A review of research 1990–2000. *Annual Review of Sex Research, 12,* 242–287.

Warr, D. J., & Pyett, P. M. (1999). Difficult relations: Sex work, love and intimacy. *Sociology of Health & Illness, 21,* 290–309. https://doi.org/10.1111/1467-9566.00157.

Weatherall, A., & Priestley, A. (2001). A feminist discourse analysis of sex 'work'. *Feminism & Psychology, 11,* 323–340. https://doi.org/10.1177/0959353501011003005.

Widom, C., & Kuhns, J. B. (1996). Childhood victimization and subsequent risk for promiscuity, prostitution, and teenage pregnancy: A prospective study. *American Journal of Public Health, 86,* 1607–1612. https://doi.org/10.2105/ajph.86.11.1607.

Williamson, C., & Folaron, G. (2003). Understanding the experiences of street level prostitutes. *Qualitative Social Work, 2,* 271–287. https://doi.org/10.1177/14733250030023004.

Wilson, H. W., & Widom, C. S. (2010). The role of youth problem behaviors in the path from child abuse and neglect to prostitution: A prospective examination. *Journal of Research in Adolescence, 20,* 210–236. https://doi.org/10.1111/j.1532-7795.2009.00624.x.

Wu, N. S., Schairer, L. C., Dellor, E., & Grella, C. (2010). Childhood trauma and health outcomes in adults with comorbid substance abuse and mental health disorders. *Addictive Behaviors, 35,* 68–71. https://doi.org/10.1016/j.addbeh.2009.09.003.

Chapter 3
Contextual Factors: Sources of Stress and How Women Cope

In general terms, stress is a person's response to adversity, demand, or challenge in his or her environment. Stress can be physiological or psychological, though it is the latter form of stress that is the focus of this chapter. Lazarus (1966, 1993) identified different types of psychological stress, including *harm,* which refers to psychological damage that has taken place; *threat,* which refers to the anticipation of harm that may be imminent; and *challenge,* which refers to stress resulting from difficult demands that people feel confident about overcoming through the use of coping resources. Stress has been examined at length in the psychological literature, with major topics including occupational stress, relationship stress, and Post-traumatic Stress Disorder (PTSD).

Consistent with the diathesis-stress model (e.g., Ingram & Luxton, 2005), the experience of stress can trigger the expression of personal predispositional vulnerabilities, resulting in mental health concerns. With this understanding, the current chapter focuses on the sources of stress that women face when they sell sex, with the goal of increasing understanding regarding women's experiences as well as increasing insight into the potential triggers for mental health concerns (discussed further in Chap. 4). We begin by reviewing some particular ways in which the activity of selling sex can be stressful. We then explore a number of contextual factors related to commercial sex, including how various locations relate to the degree of stressors experienced, this includes factors such as the legal status of selling sex within the territory worked and the particular venue or setting in which women sell sex. We also focus on the contextual stressors of social stigma in relation to the concept of *dirty work* and the experience of physical and sexual violence. Finally, we review what the literature has to offer in terms of understanding relevant coping strategies and mechanisms that women employ to reduce stress.

E. Krumrei Mancuso and B. E. Postlethwaite, *Women Who Sell Sex*,
https://doi.org/10.1007/978-3-030-47027-2_3

Stress Associated with the Activity of Selling Sex

Some research has focused on how the activity of selling sex elicits stress. Brewis and Linstead (2000) described that the sexual encounter itself may be frightening and risky. However, they emphasized that this is only one of many components of selling sex that contributes to stress. The sex acts often comprise only a small portion of the work shift. For example, women working in brothels spend extensive time waiting for customers between encounters, which can be extremely tedious; yet, the unpredictability of when customers will arrive means the women must remain vigilant at all times. Thus, the women spend a great deal of time waiting, yet not being able to relax or focus on anything else. This means their workday cycles through being "boring, terrifying, unpredictable, disgusting, and risky", which can be quite taxing, psychologically (Brewis & Linstead, 2000, p. 88). Parallels exist for women engaged in street-level work, where time between customers is spent trying to procure customers, with associated safety risks.

Another source of stress related to selling sex involves emotional strain. A phenomenon in service professions is that workers exert substantial *emotional labor* to satisfy customers (Ashforth & Humphrey, 1993; Grandey, 2000; Hochschild, 1983), which often involves modifying one's natural emotional expression by enhancing, faking, or suppressing it (Grandey, 2000). This idea can be applied to selling sex, as well. Women who sell sex often need to maintain emotional distance from customers but are simultaneously required to seem interested and affectionate (Seib, Dunne, Fischer, & Najman, 2012). Similarly, women selling sex may find certain customers to be unattractive or even repulsive. If they accept these customers, they must suppress their feelings to create the appearance of genuine attraction, liking, or connection. Constructing such illusions requires the regulation of emotions, which increases physiological demands and can thereby result in stress (Gross, 1998).

A number of scholars have argued that psychological distress experienced by women who sell sex cannot be reduced solely to the nature of the work itself, but that stress also results from a number of contextual factors, such as social stigma (e.g., Comte, 2014; Vanwesenbeeck, 2001). Likewise, some women who sell sex have indicated that their experience of violence is far more stressful than the activity of selling sex (Suresh, Furr, & Srikrishnan, 2009). Next, we will explore the major contextual factors that contribute to stress among women who sell sex. For further reading, Arnold and Barling (2003) provided an in-depth review of occupational stress in the context of commercial sex.

Context Matters: Sources of Stress

In reviewing contextual sources of stress for women who sell sex, it is important to note that the nature and severity of stressors will differ depending on the location in which women sell sex. On a macro level, this includes the country in which selling sex takes place, with the associated legal climate. On a micro level, this includes the specific venue(s) within which a woman sells sex.

Legal Status

The legal status of selling sex varies considerably by country, state/territory, and municipality. Further, the legal status of selling sex is far from static in many jurisdictions (Arnold & Barling, 2003). Laws and policies continue to change along with societal shifts in attitudes toward the sale of sex. Governments have taken three general policy approaches toward the sale of sex: criminalization, legalization, and decriminalization. In some countries, selling sex is illegal throughout the country. Often, related activities such as buying sex, pimping, or operating a brothel are also illegal. Some of the research reviewed in this book comes from countries where selling sex is illegal, including: China, South Korea, South Africa, and Thailand (although, some of these countries fall under *de facto decriminalization*, as described below). We also review research from countries where the sale of sex is legal, such as in Canada, England, Germany, the Netherlands, and Switzerland. Under *legalization*, the sale of sex is allowed, but typically regulated to some degree. Regulation efforts may include licensing, taxation, zoning restrictions, worker registration, and required health checks. Additionally, certain associated activities are often illegal. For example, in Canada, selling sex is legal, but buying sex is illegal. In England, both buying and selling sex are legal, but other activities are criminalized, including exploitation of those who sell sex, managing a brothel, and buying or selling sex in public. Decriminalization involves the removal of criminal penalties for selling sex. This is the case, for example, in New Zealand. *Full decriminalization* removes criminal penalties and leaves the sale of sex unregulated, with the exception of child prostitution, which remains illegal. Other variants include *partial decriminalization*, where criminal penalties for selling sex are reduced, and *de facto decriminalization*, where criminal penalties against selling sex exist, but are not enforced.

In a number of countries, the legal status of selling sex differs by location. For example, selling sex is criminalized throughout the United States, with the exception of certain rural counties in Nevada, where licensed brothels are permitted. In Australia, the status ranges between illegal, legal, and decriminalized, depending on the state. Similarly, in Mexico, selling sex is legal by federal law, but each state can enact and enforce laws about selling sex.

An in-depth review of the legal statuses of the sale of sex is beyond the scope of this volume and can be found within the literature (e.g., Platt et al., 2018; Weitzer, 2010, 2012). What is relevant to this chapter is the understanding that the legal status of selling sex is a contextual factor that can influence the degree of stress experienced by women who sell sex. Women who sell sex in areas where this is criminalized are continually subject to the possibility of detection, arrest, prosecution, and incarceration. They may also lack full access to the justice system or they may be subjected to harassment, intimidation, or sexual coercion by police. Among migrant women, this may be the case even in countries where selling sex is legal, if their immigration status prevents them from working or the location has a specific ban on non-residents selling sex.

Arnold and Barling (2003) considered the legal context of selling sex as a moderator of the stressor-strain relationship. That is, in response to equivalent levels of stress, women may experience greater negative strain in contexts where selling sex is prohibited. In addition, the legal climate surrounding the sale of sex can interact with other stressors, such as social stigma. Some have argued that it is impossible for the social stigma associated with selling sex to be erased in contexts where selling sex is criminalized (Thompson, 2000).

Venues

When it comes to understanding the context surrounding the sale of sex and the associated stressors, it is important to consider the specific environments or venues where research data were collected. A distinction is commonly made between outdoor or street-based work and indoor venues. The terms *outdoor* and *indoor* most commonly refer to where a commercial sex transaction originates rather than where it is consummated. For example, a woman may solicit a customer from a street corner, truck stop, or park, but subsequently go to a less public place such as the customer's car or a nearby motel to have sex. In contrast, sex may be sold indoors from venues such as brothels, massage parlors, night clubs, and private apartments. Sex that is sold indoors is often less visible than street-based sales. It may even go unnoticed by those who are not specifically looking for it. This is especially the case for commercial sex exchanges that are advertised and facilitated via the Internet.

Weitzer (2007, p. 28) has argued that indoor and outdoor work differ sharply from one another and that "many of the problems associated with 'prostitution' are actually concentrated in street prostitution and much less evident in the indoor sector." Weitzer (2009, Table 1) provided a typology of selling sex ranging from the activities of call girls to streetwalkers. According to the typology, call girls charge high prices, experience little to no exploitation by third parties, have a low risk of violent victimization, and have no impact on the community. In contrast, streetwalkers charge low prices, have a high likelihood of being victimized by third parties, have a very high risk of violent victimization, and have adverse impact on the community. Indeed, the experiences of a woman who sells sex on the street in a high-crime area (an outdoor venue) will necessarily be quite different from those of a high-end escort who operates from a luxury hotel (an indoor venue).

In understanding this distinction, it is important to note that some research, seemingly by design, employs the language of street-level work to identify precisely those situations that are risky, impoverished, or problematic, regardless of whether the sex transaction actually originated outdoors or elsewhere, such as on the internet, in crack houses, or certain types of massage parlors. This can create somewhat of an artificial distinction in the research literature between the nature of selling sex indoors and outdoors, that is more accurately based on researchers' preconceived notions about levels of risk, than about the literal indoor versus outdoor context in which sex is sold. Furthermore, we caution the reader that even within one category of venue, there may be significant variations in structure, management, safety, compensation, and stressors. For example, a small rural brothel in Nevada bears little resemblance to a large urban brothel in India, apart from the fact that both offer sex for sale indoors. It is important to keep such distinctions in mind when considering the stressors reviewed in this chapter.

Dirty Work and Social Stigma

Opinion polls about selling sex are mostly dominated by themes surrounding legality, rather than perceptions of selling sex, itself. As an exception, a YouGov (2016) poll in the United States indicated that the majority of Americans (56%) believe it is morally wrong to accept money for sex—with stronger endorsement of this opinion among women than men (YouGov, 2016). Comparative studies of European countries have examined views of the morality of buying (rather than selling) sex, with an indication that individuals in countries where the purchase of sex is criminalized are less tolerant toward buying sex compared to individuals living in countries where the purchase of sex is legal (Jonsson & Jakobsson, 2017).

Research examining perceptions of selling sex compared to other work is dated. In an early study of occupational prestige in the United States (Smith, 1943), high school and college students rated the status of 100 different occupations. The results revealed that "street prostitute" was the least prestigious occupation of all jobs considered. In another study conducted in the United States during the 1970s, drug addicts and previously incarcerated offenders rated the prestige of various legal (e.g., doctor, teacher, factory worker) and illegal (e.g., loan shark, prostitute, drug dealer) occupations (Matsueda, Gartner, Piliavin, & Polakowski, 1992). Among the illegal occupations, prostitute was ranked as being less prestigious than that of gambler, loan shark, or counterfeiter, but more prestigious than that of drug dealer, pimp, or purse snatcher.

Dirty Work

Research on *dirty work* and *stigma* offers some insight into the particular reasons that selling sex tends to be held in low esteem. Sociologist Hughes (1951, p. 319) proposed that work may be considered *dirty* for several reasons:

> It may be simply physically disgusting. It may be a symbol of degradation, something that wounds one's dignity. Finally, it may be dirty work in that it in some way goes counter to the more heroic of our moral conceptions.

That is, *dirty work* refers to activities or occupations that are tainted physically, socially, or morally (Hughes, 1958). More recently, Ashforth, Kreiner, and colleagues have expanded on the ideas proposed by Hughes (1951, 1958) by examining dirty work in considerable depth (e.g., Ashforth & Kreiner, 1999, 2014a, b; Kreiner, Ashforth, & Sluss, 2006).

Ashforth and Kreiner (1999, p. 415) maintained that *physically tainted* work involves contact with "garbage, death, effluent and so on… or is thought to be performed under particularly noxious or dangerous conditions." Examples of physically tainted occupations include butcher, janitor, funeral director, and firefighter. *Socially tainted* work involves contact with stigmatized individuals or groups or "where the worker appears to have a servile relationship to others." Examples of socially tainted occupations include police detective, social worker, butler, and maid. Finally, *morally tainted* work is generally regarded as "sinful or of dubious virtue… or where the worker is thought to employ methods that are deceptive, intrusive, confrontational, or that otherwise defy norms of civility." Examples of morally tainted work include exotic dancer, psychic, bill collector, and telemarketer.

Although some degree of dirty work exists in all occupations (Hughes, 1958), some occupations are viewed as dirtier than others. According to Ashforth and Kreiner (2014b), the dirtiest of jobs often involve moral taint, or involve a combination of multiple taints. A small number of especially dirty occupations are characterized by all three taints (moral, physical, and social), with Ashforth and Kreiner (2014b) offering prostitutes as an example, along with other occupations such as executioner and bounty hunter. Given that the presence of taint adversely impacts occupational prestige (Ashforth & Kreiner, 1999), it is not surprising that the general public does not view selling sex as a desirable occupation. However, Ashforth and Kreiner (2014a) noted that changing social views have resulted in less negative views of some morally tainted occupations. For example, drawing upon the World Values Study, Weitzer (2012, 2018) has pointed out that in countries where selling sex is legal, attitudes about selling sex are more tolerant than in countries where it is illegal. The concept of dirty work also provides a foundation for understanding *social stigma*, which we review next.

Social Stigma

Weitzer (2018) has called stigma one of the most important problems in sex work. This is seen in the empirical literature. For example, in a study of women selling sex in Nigeria, social stigma was the second largest concern noted, and it was experienced by over three-quarters of the sample (Popoola, 2013).

Sociologist Erving Goffman defined stigma as an attribute that is deeply discrediting to its possessor (Goffman, 1963). Stigmas are relational in nature—a particular attribute, such as selling sex, is not discrediting in and of itself, rather it becomes so only in the context of a relationship between social actors. Compared to an actor that is perceived as *normal*, a stigmatized individual or group is considered tainted, deficient, and lower in status. There is wide consensus that selling sex is highly stigmatized work, though the nature and severity of the stigma can vary according to context (e.g., country, venue, legal status; Jonsson & Jakobsson, 2017; Weitzer, 2018).

Stigmas apply not only to selling sex itself, but to the women who do this work. In some cases, the persons who are associated with women who sell sex also encounter stigma. This *courtesy stigma* can apply to the family members and friends of women who sell sex, as well as to researchers (Hammond & Kingston, 2014; Irvine, 2015) and those who provide services to women who sell sex (Phillips, Benoit, Hallgrimsdottir, & Vallance, 2012). Men who buy sex also encounter stigma (Hammond, 2015; Neal, 2018), though to a lesser degree than women who sell it.

Sources of Stigma

Benoit and colleagues attributed the stigma associated with selling sex to sources at three levels: macro, meso, and micro (Benoit, Jansson, Smith, & Flagg, 2018). At the macro level, stigmas may result from laws, regulations, and policies as well as from stereotypical depictions made by the media. At the meso level, the justice and health care systems may perpetuate stigma against women who sell sex. For example, police may abuse their power through excessive force, unlawful arrests, or solicitation of bribes or sexual favors. Similarly, health care systems may discriminate against, or deny care to, women who sell sex. Weitzer (2018, p. 725) has argued that anti-prostitution organizations are a meso-level source of stigma because he believes these "powerful, well-organized interest groups are committed not only to blocking any normalization of commercial sex, but also to *perpetuating and intensifying* stigmatization." At the micro level, sources of stigma include members of the public, who may harass or demean women who sell sex, as well as women who sell sex themselves, who may distance themselves from other women who sell sex under less favorable circumstances (such as on the street) or who have more discrediting characteristics than themselves (e.g., substance abuse or status as a racial minority; Benoit et al., 2018).

Degree of Stigma

People may have more compassion toward women they view as victims of human trafficking. In contrast, they may stigmatize to a greater extent women who *choose* to sell sex, because these women violate gender norms and stereotypes about female sexuality (Shaver, 1994). Further, the level of stigma experienced by women selling sex may vary depending on where and how sex is sold. For example, women selling sex on the street encounter greater societal judgment than women engaged in high-end escort work. In part, this may be due to the fact that women selling sex on the street are considerably more visible to the public than those who sell sex indoors. In addition, this illustrates how social factors such as socioeconomic status can interact with the choice to sell sex with regard to the degree of stigma experienced.

A small amount of quantitative research has focused on what characteristics of selling sex are associated with experiencing more or less social stigma. Among women selling sex in the Dominican Republic, numerous factors were found to be predictive of the women feeling devaluation by others because of selling sex (Rael, 2015). More time spent selling sex was a predictor of experiencing stigma from one's community. Specifically, each hour spent selling sex per week was associated with a 1% increase in feelings of devaluation from one's community. On the other hand, working independently, nationality, and living with children were all protective factors. The odds of perceiving stigma from one's community were 66% lower for women who sold sex independently compared to women employed at a venue, 65% lower for Haitians compared to Dominicans and other nationalities, and 37% lower for women whose children lived with them. Living with one's children was not only a protective factor for stigma from one's community, but also for stigma from one's family. The odds of feeling devalued by one's family members were 40% lower for mothers who sold sex and lived with their children compared to mothers who sold sex but did not have their minor children in their household. Education was an additional protective factor, with the odds of feeling stigma from one's family decreasing 12% for each additional year of education achieved. Finally, the odds of feeling stigma from one's family for selling sex were 78% higher for women who provided the primary economic support for their households. Although this finding may appear counterintuitive, Rael (2015) suggested it might be explained by the fact that in the Dominican Republic, women earning income challenges gender ideologies and thereby heightens the degree of stigma experienced. Overall, these findings illustrate that many factors are related to the degree to which women who sell sex experience social stigma. In this cultural context examined, the flexibility of working for oneself, spending less time selling sex, greater anonymity associated with being a migrant sex worker, and adhering to traditional notions about mothering seemed to be protective factors from stigma related to selling sex. Among this sample, many women selling sex and their families considered commercial sex to be an important income-generating activity to be used as an advancement strategy (Rael, 2015). Therefore, women selling sex in other parts of the world may experience more stigma from family members than those who participated in this particular study.

Additional research has indicated that venue management can also impact the level of stigma experienced by a women who sells sex within establishments. A study from China indicated that experiencing more trust, communication, and support in relation to the manager of the commercial sex venue is associated with experiencing less stigma, even when controlling demographic characteristics, alcohol and drug use, and the experience of partner violence (Zhang, Li, Hong, Su, & Zhou, 2014).

Multiple Stigmas

Women who sell sex may face additional stigmas outside of their involvement in commercial sex (Chapkis, 2018; Sanders, 2018). For example, women who sell sex may also encounter stigma due to gender, race, social class, health status, substance use, and immigration status. Thus, it is very possible to have a complex, multi-layering of stigmas that is difficult to untangle and equally difficult to address. Researchers have argued that any attempt to address the stigma associated with selling sex in isolation is likely to be ineffective due to the presence and power of other stigmas.

The Effects of Stigma

Stigma can have wide-ranging effects on women who sell sex, including the impacts of associated denigrating attitudes and behaviors from others, such as receiving insults, being called derogatory names or labels, being denied social rights or health care, and as a result, feeling socially outcast (see Benoit et al., 2018 for a review). Stigma can even impact women's most personal relationships, as illustrated by a qualitative study of women in Australia, where social stigma attached to selling sex was a barrier to the women's partners in offering support and understanding within the relationship (Bellhouse, Crebbin, Fairley, & Bilardi, 2015).

In addition to experiencing direct effects of stigma, social stigma can also lead to secondary difficulties, such as women feeling restricted about telling others what they do for a living (Bellhouse et al., 2015). This can have numerous ill effects. It often results in women maintaining dual identities in an attempt to keep their involvement in commercial sex hidden and they may restrict themselves to a very closed social circle in which other women who sell sex become their main peer group. In such cases, the women's worlds become circumscribed by their involvement in selling sex (see Brewis & Linstead, 2000). In addition, social stigma can form a barrier to seeking mental health care for women who sell sex (Rayson & Alba, 2019; Zehnder, Mutschler, Rössler, Rufer, & Rüsch, 2019). The effect of stigma can remain a source of stress even after women transition out of selling sex, since there is a continual threat that their previous involvement in selling sex may be discovered by others.

Beyond contributing to stress, the direct and indirect effects of stigma can relate to other mental health concerns, including anxiety, depression, and suicidal thinking. In a study from China, the more social stigma women selling sex perceived, the more likely they were to experience depression, suicidal ideation, and suicide attempts (Hong et al., 2010). In another study, worries about being known by family as a sex worker were predictive of suicidal ideation and suicide attempts among women selling sex in rural China (Hong, Li, Fang, & Zhao, 2007). Finally, in a study conducted in the United States and Canada, researchers compared the relationship between depression and discrimination attributable to stigma in three occupational populations: sex workers, hair stylists, and restaurant servers (Benoit, McCarthy, & Jansson, 2015). Compared to hair stylists and restaurant servers, those who sold sex experienced higher levels of discrimination and displayed more depression and less self-worth. They found that discrimination, a measure of stigma, mediated the relationship between selling sex and depression. We should note that this study included men in both the sex work (13.9%) and non-sex work (23.9%) groups; despite this, we include it in our review given that that it is one of few quantitative studies to examine stigma and mental health outcomes among those who sell sex. Additional strengths of this study include the use of comparison groups, a validated depression scale, and robust control variables.

Managing and Reducing Stigma

Some women attempt to prevent stigma by limiting disclosures about their involvement in commercial sex. Disclosure approaches can range from complete concealment, to selective or partial disclosure, to full disclosure or *coming out* (Benoit et al., 2018; Koken, 2012). Besides this, many women use role separation, disengagement, and distancing to manage stigmatization about selling sex. These approaches are covered in the coping section of this chapter. For an in-depth review of stigma management, see Benoit et al. (2018).

Weitzer (2018) noted that the great majority of work on stigma encountered by those who sell sex has focused on managing stigma rather than reducing or eliminating it. In contrast to managing stigma, which is done at the individual level, reducing or eliminating stigma requires collective or institutional action. Recent efforts in this regard have adopted a harm reduction approach centered around mobilizing groups of women who sell sex in an effort to combat stigma that can serve as a barrier to health interventions (e.g., Biradavolu, Blankenship, Jena, & Dhungana, 2012; Scambler & Paolo, 2008).

Physical and Sexual Violence

The experience of violence and the threat of violence are both major sources of stress for women who sell sex. Violence is a key concern that drives discussion about policy and outreach surrounding the sale of sex. For this reason, a great amount of research has focused on this topic, allowing us to cover it in greater depth. Specifically, we will explore the frequency, nature, and sources of violence experienced by women who sell sex, examine what the predictors are of experiencing more or less violence in commercial sex contexts, review how the experience of violence relates to selling sex, and consider how violence relates to mental health.

Sources of Violence

The sources of violence faced by women who sell sex are diverse. Of interest in the research literature has been violence experienced from customers. However, women who sell sex also encounter violence from brothel or other venue owners or employees, pimps, strangers, and the police (e.g., Nixon, Tutty, Downe, Gorkoff, & Ursel, 2002; Odinokova, Rusakova, Urada, Silverman, & Raj, 2014; Rodriguez, Fuentes, Ramos-Lira, Gutierrez, & Ruiz, 2014; Suresh et al., 2009). Some research has even suggested that women experience more violence from other sex workers than from customers (Rodríguez et al.2014).

It is important to point out that women who sell sex experience violence not only in the context of commercial sex, but also in other aspects of their lives. Outside of selling sex, women experience violence from family, significant others, and strangers (Nixon et al., 2002). For comparison purposes, in a study of women selling sex on the street in New York City, approximately half of the women had experienced physical and/or sexual violence from customers, but a staggering 73% of the women had experienced physical or sexual abuse by an intimate partner (El-Bassel, Witte, Wada, Gilbert, & Wallace, 2001). Although, comparing rates of violence within the previous year only, indicated that violence from customers (32%) was more common than from an intimate partner (22%). This difference was attributable primarily to higher rates of sexual abuse from customers, as rates of physical abuse from customers over the previous year were similar to rates of physical abuse from intimate partners, but rates of sexual abuse were much higher from customers (22%) than from intimate partners (4%). The presence of sexual violence in women's personal lives is supported by another, smaller study of women who sold sex on the street, among whom 75% had been raped by one or more customers and 63% had been raped in contexts outside of selling sex. Thus, when considering the mental health outcomes of experiencing violence, it is important to realize that violence experienced in the context of selling sex may be compounded by violence experienced in other settings, which may have even predated entry into selling sex. Text Box 3.1 further explores research on the overall links between violence and selling sex.

Text Box 3.1 Violence and Selling Sex: The Chicken Versus Egg Dilemma

Many studies have indicated links between selling sex and the experience of violence. This relationship has not necessarily been shown for emotional abuse (Gilchrist, Gruer, & Atkinson, 2005), but has been consistently found for adulthood (Gilchrist et al., 2005; Perdue et al., 2012) and lifetime prevalence (Molitor, Ruiz, Klausner, & McFarland, 2000; Urada et al., 2014) of physical and sexual abuse, with those who have experienced violence being up to six times more likely to sell sex than those who have not experienced violence (Molitor et al., 2000). The links seem to be strongest for those who have experienced violence that is more traumatic. For example, in one study, victims of multiple-assault attacks, like gang rapes, were more likely to have sold sex after their assaults than victims of single assault rapes (Campbell, Ahrens, Sefl, & Clark, 2003).

Some strengths in the literature examining links between violence and selling sex are that it is representative of a number of different countries, including the Philippines (Urada et al., 2014), Scotland (Gilchrist et al., 2005), and the United States (Campbell et al., 2003; Molitor et al., 2000; Potterat et al., 1985) and that attempts have been made at representative sampling. Studies have recruited women from random samplings of bars and spas (Urada et al., 2014), representative zip codes of cities (Campbell et al., 2003) and randomly selected dwellings in low-income neighborhoods (Molitor et al., 2000). Some research has also made use of matched comparison designs (Potterat et al., 1985). Further, most studies controlled for relevant personal characteristics among participants, such as age, race, education, partner status, employment, and income.

Among research conducted in the United States, a prevalent theme has been that experiencing intimate partner violence is associated with selling sex or trading sex for drugs or other goods (El-Bassel, Simoni, Cooper, Gilbert, & Schilling, 2001). For example, in one study, women who had ever sold sex were more likely to be in a violent relationship at the time of the study (Perdue et al., 2012). In addition, a small study assessing women selling sex and a matched comparison group found many similarities between the two groups of women, including similar levels of childhood physical and sexual abuse, but found that a much larger percentage of those selling sex reported being abused by a spouse or lover (Potterat, Phillips, Rothenberg, & Darrow, 1985). Research has indicated that women who have experienced intimate partner violence are more than four times as likely to trade sex for money, food, shelter, or drugs than those who have not had a violent partner (DeHart, Lynch, Belknap, Dass-Brailsford, & Green, 2014). However, a confounding issue in the research on intimate partner violence is that much of this work has not ruled out the possibility that the violence reported is attributable to a pimp. Meaning, it is possible, though unclear to what extent, the link between intimate partner violence and selling sex can be explained on the basis of violent partners directly coercing women to engage in commercial sex. Another limitation in the research on intimate partner violence and selling sex is that it has tended to drawn on populations that are vulnerable for reasons other than selling sex, such as women who have a drug addiction (El-Bassel et al., 2001; Gilchrist et al., 2005), sexually transmitted disease (Potterat et al., 1985), or criminal record (DeHart et al., 2014; Perdue et al., 2012).

Additional problematic limitations in the body of literature examining links between violence and selling sex is that many of these studies did not assess the time ordering of violence in relation to entry into commercial sex. Thus, it is not always clear whether experiencing violence increases entry into commercial sex, or whether women who sell sex are more likely to experience violence, whether during or outside of the sale of sex. Even when time-ordering is reported, causality cannot be assumed. Despite this, some women personally attribute their selling sex to the violence they experienced. For example, among rape survivors who sold sex, 75% of women indicated they believed their selling sex was directly related to having being raped (Campbell et al., 2003).

Other mechanisms may also be at work, such as psychological distress. It is clear that physical and sexual abuse in adulthood are predictive of more mental health concerns among samples of women who sell sex (Gilchrist et al., 2005) and that women who sell sex after being raped show higher levels of psychological distress than women who do not sell sex after being raped (Campbell et al., 2003). Consequently, one hypothesis is that psychological distress may mediate links between violence and selling sex.

Clearly, even though causality cannot be established in either direction between violence and selling sex on the basis of this research, the experience of violence among women who sell sex, whether this occurs prior to, during, or outside of the sale of sex, is a relevant contributor to the diathesis-stress model of mental health for women who sell sex.

Rates of Violence

The rate of violence experienced by women while selling sex differs widely within the literature. Some researchers have pointed out that some women sell sex without experiencing any violence (O'Doherty, 2011). Across studies, percentages of women who have experienced physical violence while selling sex tend to range from around 25% on the low end (Surratt, Inciardi, Kurtz, & Kiley, 2004) to 90% on the high end (Farley, Lynne, & Cotton, 2005) and percentages of women who have experienced sexual violence while selling sex range from around 13% on the low end (Suratt et al., 2004) to 94% on the high end (Miller & Schwartz, 1995). There are numerous factors that might account for this drastic range. First, the literature indicates that levels of violence differ on the basis of the country in which sex is sold. These differences could be due to levels of social stigma directed toward selling sex, in part on the basis of the legal status of selling sex (see previous chapter sections on this) and differences in cultural norms surrounding violence toward those who sell sex (e.g., Suratt et al., 2004).

Regardless of country, rates of violence also seem to differ on the basis of the particular context in which sex is sold (Weitzer, 2009). Although violence occurs in both indoor and outdoor venues, a prevalent theme in the literature is that rates of violence seem higher when women sell sex on the street rather than indoors (e.g., Krumrei-Mancuso, 2017; O'Doherty 2011; Seib et al., 2012; Shaver, 2005; Whittaker & Hart, 1996). For example, in a study of women selling sex in three major British cities, working outdoors rather than indoors was associated with higher levels of violence by customers (Church, Henderson, Barnard, & Hart, 2001). In this study, 81% of women working outdoors had ever experienced violence from customers, compared to 48% of those working indoors. Half of those working outdoors reported violence by customers in the past six months, compared to half this rate for those working indoors (50.4% outdoors versus 25.6% indoors). This outdoor-indoor distinction was a stronger predictor of violence than other factors such as drug use, age of entry and duration of involvement in commercial sex, and the city in which the women worked (Church et al., 2001).

A major contributor to the differing rates of violence between street and indoor contexts is access to safety strategies, such as those offered by the collective nature of an indoor venue (Sanders & Campbell, 2007). Those who work in brothels and other indoor establishments have other workers and staff members nearby. For example, a receptionist can screen customers for intoxication or suspicious behavior (Sanders & Campbell, 2007). Along these lines, research from China has indicated that having a close relationship with the manager of one's commercial sex venue is predictive of experiencing less violence from customers as well as significant others (Zhang et al., 2014). In addition, many indoor venues have security cameras in general areas and alarm buttons in each room. Safety measures are also taken by women who work independently indoors. For example, in the UK, a sex worker organization, the National Ugly Mugs, operates an online service that provides safety alerts and facilitates confidential reporting of violent incidents and assaults (Sanders, Connelly, & King, 2016).

Access to safety measures is influenced not only by the literal distinction between indoor and outdoor activities, but also by factors such as the socioeconomic situation of the women and the legal status of selling sex. This is illustrated by the fact that an exception to the indoor-outdoor discrepancy in rates of violence is found in crack houses, rife with poverty, addiction, and illegal activities, where much more physical and sexual abuse from customers takes place than in other indoor locations (El-Bassel, Witte, Wada, Gilbert, & Wallace, 2001). In general, lower socioeconomic status and greater social isolation are associated with experiencing more violence when selling sex. For example, among women who sold sex on the street in New York, not having an intimate partner in one's personal life, being homeless, not having a source of income outside of selling sex, and having been incarcerated in the past year were all associated with a greater likelihood of being physically and sexually abused by customers (El-Bassel et al., 2001).

Another consideration is that street-level work, itself, is rarely legal, even in countries where selling sex indoors is legal. Therefore, those working on the street will not only lack access to general safety measures, but may, to a certain extent, lack access to protection from police. For example, in a study from Australia, women who sold sex illegally, mostly on the streets, were more likely to have been recently raped or assaulted by a customer compared to women working legally indoors (Seib et al., 2012). At times, those working outdoors may even face violence from police (Odinokova et al., 2014). Protection from such violence is a major motivational factor for selling sex under someone else's management, as those working under pimps and madams are less likely to report a history of police sexual coercion (Odinokova et al., 2014).

Notably, there have been some efforts to improve safety in outdoor venues. As one example, in 2013, the city of Zurich constructed drive-in sex boxes to provide a safer environment for street-based sex transactions (Folkes, 2013). These outdoor booths featured security patrols and alarm buttons as well as on-site social services. Similar efforts have been undertaken in other cities.

Outcomes of Violence

Although rare studies have found no evidence that physical assault while selling sex is associated with prevalence of PTSD (Roxburgh et al., 2006), a majority of studies have linked violence experienced while selling sex to mental health concerns, including PTSD and depression (e.g., Farley & Barkan, 1998; Farley et al., 2003; Vanwesenbeeck, de Graaf, van Zessen, Straver, & Visser, 1993). As may be expected, women who experience more violence while selling sex display higher levels of PTSD and depression than those who experience less violence while selling sex (Rössler et al., 2010; Suresh et al., 2009). These findings hold with regard to sexual violence. The experience of rape and adult sexual assault while engaged in commercial sex have been associated with a greater prevalence and severity of PTSD (Farley & Barkan, 1998; Roxburgh et al., 2006). We discuss these mental health outcomes in more depth in Chap. 4.

Violence is associated not only with mental health symptoms, but also with death among women who sell sex. The most comprehensive research on homicide among women selling sex has been conducted in high-income countries such as the United States (Brewer et al., 2006; Quinet, 2011), Canada (Beuaregard & Martineau, 2012), and the United Kingdom (Cunningham, Sanders, Platt, Grenfell, & Macioti, 2018; Salfati, James, & Ferguson, 2008). Compared to other groups, women who sell sex face a substantially increased risk of lethal violence. In their review, Brewer and colleagues (2006) reported that women who sell sex have the highest homicide victimization rate of any set of women ever studied, representing 2.7% of female homicide victims between 1982 and 2000.

A 30-year, large-scale study in the United States indicated that women who sold sex were almost 18 times more likely to be murdered than a comparison sample of women of similar age and race who did not sell sex during the same time period (Potterat et al., 2004). In fact, homicide accounted for 50% of the deaths among the sample of women selling sex, with the vast majority of these women being killed as a direct consequence of selling sex. Similarly, a 9-year prospective study of women selling sex in London found that their death rate was 12 times that of same-aged women who did not sell sex, and half of the mortality was attributable to murder (Ward, Day, & Weber, 1999). However, in the latter study, the higher death rate was not attributable to selling sex alone, but also to other factors, such as poverty, homelessness, and substance abuse. In a more recent study in the UK (Cunningham et al., 2018), the authors argued that a distinction should be made between homicides that occur while the victim is selling sex versus homicides that occur in other contexts. The former can be referred to as "occupational homicide," and classifying deaths in this manner will allow a better understanding of the circumstances surrounding homicides as well as more focused policy responses. Where data are available, the indication seems to be that the majority of homicides are committed by customers rather than pimps or other women who sell sex (Brewer et al., 2006). Moreover, it has been estimated that approximately a third of the homicides of women who sell sex are attributable to serial killers (32% between 1970 and 2009, Quinet, 2011, and 35% between 1982 and 2000, Brewer et al., 2006).

Traditionally, women engaged in street-based commercial sex have been more vulnerable due to the fact that they often work alone, at night, and in high-risk environments (Quinet, 2011). The same factors raise the risk for homicide among people employed outside of commercial sex, such as police officers, taxi drivers, and retail clerks (Kraus, 1987). However, Cunningham and colleagues (2018) found that between 2010 and 2016, more homicides were committed against women who worked indoors (59%, n = 10) versus on the street (41%, n = 7). This differed from previous decades, in which the majority (85%) of homicides had been committed against women who were street-based. This change could be due to the growth of Internet-based methods of selling sex and, thereby, the significant decline of the street-based sale of sex in the United Kingdom (Sanders, Scoular, Campbell, Pitcher, & Cunningham, 2018).

Drug and alcohol use seem to be relevant factors in understanding the risk of homicide for women who sell sex. Brewer et al. (2008) noted that there was an increase in homicides among both women who sell sex and their customers beginning in the late 1980 and early 1990s, which could potentially be attributed to a rise in the use of crack cocaine. Crack cocaine use can result in increased vulnerability and increased aggression, both of which can contribute to the likelihood of homicide. For example, data from homicides of women related to selling sex in 1988 in thirty-three urban United States counties showed 82% (14/17) of victims were under the influence of cocaine at the time of the homicide (Brewer et al., 2006, Table 7). Similarly, 74% of victims of homicides related to selling sex (51/69) between 1988 and mid-2000 were under the influence of cocaine (Brewer et al., 2006, Table 7). Likewise, Salfati and colleagues (2008) found that 93.9% (31/33) of female homicide victims who had been selling sex in the UK between 1990 and 2001 had been involved in some form of substance abuse (alcohol, drugs, or solvents). However, the direct role, if any, that substances played in their deaths was not reported.

Factors That Contribute to Violence Against Women Who Sell Sex

We are not arguing that physical and sexual assault and harassment are unique to women who sell sex. These factors form significant stressors in a variety of jobs (e.g., Shaver, 2005). For example, those in law enforcement, security guards, and bartenders experience relatively high rates of workplace violence (Harrell, 2011). However, given the focus of this book is on the experiences of women who sell sex, it is worth considering the factors that might uniquely underlie the prevalence of violence toward this group of individuals.

Based on qualitative interviews with sixteen women who sold sex on the street, Miller and Schwartz (1995) have argued that rape myths fuel violence against women who sell sex. Specifically, the common belief that women who sell sex are publicly available for male consumption has led to the myth that these women are "unrapeable" (p. 10, 11), meaning that they have given up their right to consent and, therefore, are open territory for assault. This is poignantly illustrated by a case in which an Australian man convicted of raping a woman who sold sex received a lighter sentence because the judge believed the victim "was less psychologically harmed by the rape" than would have been the case if she were a "chaste woman" (Scutt, 1994, p. 346). The fact that such thinking is present in judicial systems illustrates that rape myths are a social problem, not a thinking style exclusive to men who buy sex. In fact, male customers of women who sell sex are not, in general, more likely to endorse rape myths than other samples of men (Monto, 2010). In his work with over 1,000 customers, Monto (2010) has argued that most men who buy sex do not hold views that justify violence against women who sell sex. Rather, when violence occurs, it seems to be the general, social devaluation of women who sell sex that allows this violence against them to be ignored in society. For example, qualitative interviews with women engaged in street-level commercial sex have indicated that if they became victims of crimes, they were largely ignored by the justice system (Miller & Schwartz, 1995). Women who sell sex, along with drug users, migrants, and the homeless, are part of a marginalized group that Egger (2002) referred to as "the less-dead." Because these highly stigmatized individuals are seen as having less valuable lives than persons with higher social standing, their deaths are considered less noteworthy in society. Perpetrators may feel less guilt when committing violent or lethal acts against these individuals. Furthermore, when "less-dead" individuals become victims of homicide, fewer resources may be devoted to investigation than if the victims were more prominent members of society. As illustrated, perpetrators who are convicted of violent acts against women who sell sex may face lesser penalties than if their victim were not engaged in the commercial sex trade. All of these social conditions may contribute to the prevalence of violence against women who sell sex.

The threat of violence, the experience of violence, the lack of representation within the justice system, and the underlying social attitudes that contribute to violence can all have serious mental health implications for women who sell sex. This is relevant to helping professionals who can addressed these issues via prevention and intervention services. Specific implications for mental health professionals are discussed in Chap. 7.

Coping

Despite the serious stressors faced by women who sell sex, not much research has focused on how these women cope. Only a small number of studies have examined various strategies and techniques that women who sell sex use to cope with stress. These techniques are typically classified as being problem-focused or emotion-focused in nature. Problem-focused coping refers to engaging in practical behaviors to try to remove or reduce a stressor. Examples include problem-solving, seeking information or assistance, or removing oneself from the stressful situation. This type of coping is often most helpful in response to situations in which the individual can exert some control over the stressor. Emotion-focused coping involves efforts to reduce one's negative emotional responses to a stressor, such as working to minimize fear, anxiety, or depression. This can be done by talking, praying, or writing about one's emotions, distracting oneself to take one's mind off of a stressor, eating, using alcohol or drugs, reframing one's thoughts about a stressor, or suppressing negative emotions. As demonstrated by the examples, particular forms of coping can be either helpful or harmful to an individual depending on their nature and the degree to which they are used, for example, exercising to distract oneself can be a useful way to cope with difficult emotions, but not if it becomes obsessive. The usefulness of coping mechanisms will also depend on context. Specifically, emotion-focused coping stands in contrast to practical ways of coping that target the cause of stress, and emotion-focused coping is therefore most beneficial when the source of stress is outside of a person's control. When individuals have the ability to address a stressor directly, problem-focused coping is usually more beneficial.

General Coping

A number of quantitative studies have assessed the extent to which women who sell sex use various commonly recognized coping strategies to manage stress in everyday living. One study examined how HIV-positive females selling sex in Nepal coped with the stress of being HIV positive (Eller & Mahat, 2003).[1] The most commonly used strategy was seeking social support (18% of sample), followed by positive

[1] Of note is that this sample included youth as young as 13 years of age, and an average age of 20 years. Therefore, this study does not fit the criteria we set for reviewing research on adults only, however, we include it here given the analyses of this study demonstrated that those above and below the median age of 19 years showed no differences in general coping styles.

reappraisal or cognitive reframing of situations (15% of sample), confrontive coping (13% of sample), distancing themselves from stressful situations (13% of sample), problem solving (12% of sample), trying to escape or avoid negative thoughts or distressing situations (11% of sample), self-controlling (10% of sample), and accepting responsibility (8% of sample). Overall, these women were more likely to rely on problem-focused coping strategies (58% of sample) than emotion-focused coping strategies (32% of sample). Of note is that this sample reported relatively low levels of stress, similar to levels reported by women in the general population. Among women who sell sex who have more mental health concerns, emotion-focused coping may be more prevalent (e.g., 56.7% of women described by Ansari, Gharraee, & Afsar-Kazerouni, 2011). However, it should also be noted that some coping instruments classify coping strategies differently with regard to designating them as problem-versus emotion-focused, making it more difficult to compare across studies.

Dalla, Xia, and Kennedy (2003) have examined what factors might be responsible for relying on different forms of coping among women who previously or currently sold sex on the street. They found that having experienced more stressful life events, such as the loss of a family member or friend, being a victim of violence, or being in trouble with the law, were each associated with more escapism (e.g., distracting from distress through food or drugs, an emotion-focused strategy) and internalizing (e.g., keeping feelings to oneself, an emotion-focused strategy), and with less seeking of assistance from others (a problem-focused strategy). This suggests that women who experience the most stress may be relying more on coping mechanisms that are ill-fitting to their situations. In contrast, they found that having a strong social network was associated with more adaptive forms of coping. Specifically, experiencing more emotional and practical support in one's close relationships were both associated with coping by taking action (e.g., doing something about one's situation, a problem-focused approach). Experiencing emotional support in one's relationships was further predictive of coping by seeking social assistance (a problem-focused approach) and experiencing practical support in relationships was associated with coping through emotional support from others (an emotion-focused approach). Although this study did not assess coping specifically with stressors related to selling sex, the findings suggest that among women who sell sex on the street, those who experience the most life stressors are also the most in need of psychoeducation and support to bolster healthy coping mechanisms. Moreover, having reliable social networks seems to be key to healthy coping, which highlights the importance of strengthening social support systems where possible among women selling sex on the street.

Coping With Selling Sex

Some studies have indicated that women generally lack strategies for coping with the stressors associated with selling sex. For example, a study of women selling sex in Nigeria indicated that simply enduring stressors associated with selling sex was a common way of responding, and was far more common than relying on counseling, prayer, or other forms of coping (Popoola, 2013). However, quite a bit of qualitative research has described in detail various ways that women cope specifically with the challenges they face while selling sex.

Given the physically intimate nature of selling sex, a common coping mechanism surrounds the need to distance, or mentally separate oneself from customers, as a form of emotional protection. Over half of a sample of women selling sex in Australia indicated that they found it quite or very difficult to mentally separate their work lives from their personal lives (Bellhouse et al., 2015). Distancing has, at times, been described in a harmful light, particularly if it is associated with disengaging in the form of depersonalization. However, Shaver (1994) has argued that distancing is a healthy coping strategy used successfully to create emotional protection for individuals in many occupations, including doctors, nurses, hospital attendants, masseurs, morticians, social workers, psychologists, flight attendants, and others. Distancing can take many different forms when selling sex. One is that women take a clinical approach to selling sex in which they respond to the customer's desires without experiencing any personal emotional or sexual interest (Sanders, 2005). A specific mechanism women may use to accomplish this is engaging an internal dialogue to stay detached while engaging in sex. Women may also differentiate work sex from personal sex in a number of different ways, such as enforcing rules (monitoring time limits, keeping certain physical acts off limits, strictly enforcing condom use, etc.). Other ways in which women engage in role separation is by playing a character with a pseudonym in interacting with customers. This is a mechanism for protecting the true self. Women have also used various methods of marking off physical space when selling sex, such as restricting the commercial sex space to particular colors in the decorating scheme or using separate linens than in daily life. For a more detailed review of the qualitative literature on distancing and role separation, see Brewis and Linstead (2000).

Another, less constructive, method of coping that has been highlighted in the literature is alcohol and drug use as a form of escape or avoidance. Women may use alcohol or drugs to numb themselves when working in unfavorable circumstances or to emotionally detach themselves from interactions with customers (Kramer, 2003; Roxburgh et al., 2006). This is consistent with what is known as the self-medication hypothesis (Khantzian, 1997), in which alcohol or drugs are used to cope with emotional or psychological pain resulting from selling sex. Both self-report descriptions of coping through alcohol and drugs and research showing that women mostly consume alcohol on days that they sell sex rather than on days off support this hypothesis, although the latter data can also result from the availability of alcohol when selling sex or the fact that women in some venues earn money by drinking with customers, in addition to providing sexual services (van Nunen, Leuridan, Van Hal, Van Damme, & Decorte, 2014). Substance use and associated disorders in relation to selling sex are examined in depth in Chap. 5.

Discussion

Sex is not sold in a vacuum; rather, it is sold in a unique social context where legal status, societal norms, particular work setting, and individual differences intersect to influence the experiences of a given woman. The prevalence of social stigma and the threat of violence are two important contextual factors that increase stress for women who sell sex.

Although stigma toward selling sex may be weakening in some areas where more liberalized attitudes toward sexual commerce have developed, it is clear that selling sex remains highly stigmatized in most locations around the globe. Women who sell sex experience pervasive and powerful stigma that can impact self-identity, stress levels, and ultimately physical and psychological health. We believe that, regardless of one's ideological stance toward selling sex, women who sell sex deserve to be treated with dignity and respect. Proponents of selling sex as legitimate work have long been vocal about the need to minimize stigma and prejudice directed toward women who sell sex. In our view, the agendas of abolitionists also benefits from decreased social stigma directed toward women who sell sex, given that research among other populations, such as racial and ethnic minorities and individuals with mental illness, has suggested that social attitudes such as stereotypes can result in self-fulfilling prophecies, reinforcing the behavior that is the target of the stereotype. Similarly, stigmas have been associated with feelings of shame, which in turn have been associated with more risky behavior, including risky sexual behavior (e.g., Stuewig et al., 2015). Consequently, reducing stigmatization may reduce harm. Thereby, every stakeholder wins when harmful stigmas are reduced.

In addition to experiencing stigma, it is clear that many (but not all) women who sell sex are exposed to physical or sexual violence either in the course of selling sex or in other contexts. Violence is typically more prevalent in certain work environments, such as on the street. However, indoor venues are not free from violence. Further, as commercial sex continues to shift indoors with the growth of the Internet, patterns of violence are shifting. Therefore, updated research is needed on indoor venues. Such research should not be limited to high income countries, rather it should examine a variety of socio-economic contexts.

Finally, much more research is needed to understand the many ways in which women who sell sex cope with life stressors, and in particular, with the stressors surrounding selling sex. It seems that women manage stress through a variety of coping strategies ranging from healthy (e.g., role separation, humor) to unhealthy (e.g., substance abuse). The limited research conducted to date on this topic suggests that precisely those women who face the most stress may be relying more on maladaptive coping mechanisms. Therefore, there is a need for psychoeducation among this community to help women understand how they can employ more adaptive forms of coping. The literature also suggests that having a reliable social network is related to drawing on helpful coping mechanisms, thus, this may pose an additional point of intervention.

References

Ansari, S., Gharraee, B., & Afsar-Kazerouni, P. (2011). Personality disorders and coping strategies in female sex-workers. *Iranian Journal of Psychiatry and Clinical Psychology, 17,* 71–75.

Arnold, K. A., & Barling, J. (2003). Prostitution: An illustration of occupational stress in 'dirty work'. In M. Dollard, H. R. Winefield, & A. H. Winefield (Eds.), *Occupational stress in the service professions* (pp. 261–280). London: CRC Press.

Ashforth, B. E., & Humphrey, R. H. (1993). Emotional labor in service roles: The influence of identity. *Academy of Management Review, 18,* 88–115. https://doi.org/10.2307/258824.

Ashforth, B. E., & Kreiner, G. E. (1999). "How can you do it?": Dirty work and the challenge of constructing a positive identity. *Academy of Management Review, 24,* 413–434. https://doi.org/10.5465/amr.1999.2202129.

Ashforth, B. E., & Kreiner, G. E. (2014a). Contextualizing dirty work: The neglected role of cultural, historical, and demographic context. *Journal of Management & Organization, 20,* 423–440. https://doi.org/10.1017/jmo.2014.38.

Ashforth, B. E., & Kreiner, G. E. (2014b). Dirty work and dirtier work: Differences in countering physical, social, and moral stigma. *Management and Organization Review, 10,* 81–108. https://doi.org/10.1111/more.12044.

Beauregard, E., & Martineau, M. (2012). A descriptive study of sexual homicide in Canada: Implications for police investigation. *International Journal of Offender Therapy and Comparative Criminology, 57,* 1454–1476. https://doi.org/10.1177/0306624X12456682.

Bellhouse, C., Crebbin, S., Fairley, C. K., & Bilardi, J. E. (2015). The impact of sex work on women's personal romantic relationships and the mental separation of their work and personal lives: A mixed-methods study. *PLoS One, 10*(10). https://doi.org/10.1371/journal.pone.0141575.

Benoit, C., McCarthy, B., & Jansson, M. (2015). Stigma, sex work, and substance use: a comparative analysis. *Sociology of Health & Illness, 37,* 437–451. https://doi.org/10.1111/1467-9566.12201.

Benoit, C., Jansson, S. M., Smith, M., & Flagg, J. (2018). Prostitution stigma and its effect on the working conditions, personal lives, and health of sex workers. *Journal of Sex Research, 55,* 457–471. https://doi.org/10.1080/00224499.2017.1393652.

Biradavolu, M. R., Blankenship, K. M., Jena, A., & Dhungana, N. (2012). Structural stigma, sex work and HIV: Contradictions and lessons learnt from a community-led structural intervention in southern India. *Journal of Epidemiology and Community Health, 66,* ii95–ii.99. https://doi.org/10.1136/jech-2011-200508.

Brewer, D. D., Dudek, J. A., Potterat, J. J., Muth, S. Q., Roberts, J. M., & Woodhouse, D. E. (2006). Extent, trends, and perpetrators of prostitution-related homicide in the United States. *Journal of Forensic Science, 51,* 1101-1108. doi:10.1111/j.1556-4029.2006.00206.x

Brewer, D. D., Dudek, J. A., Potterat, J. J., Muth, S. Q., Roberts, J. M., Jr., & Woodhouse, D. E. (2006). Extent, trends, and perpetrators of prostitution-related homicide in the United States. *Journal of Forensic Sciences, 51,* 1101–1108. https://doi.org/10.1111/j.1556-4029.2006.00206.x.

Brewis, J., & Linstead, S. (2000). 'The worst thing is the screwing' (1): Consumption and the management of identity in sex work. *Gender, Work and Organization, 7,* 84–97. https://doi.org/10.1111/1468-0432.00096.

Campbell, R., Ahrens, C. E., Sefl, T., & Clark, M. L. (2003). The relationship between adult sexual assault and prostitution: An exploratory analysis. *Violence and Victims, 18,* 299–317. https://doi.org/10.1891/vivi.2003.18.3.299.

Chapkis, W. (2018). Commentary: Response to Weitzer 'Resistance to sex work stigma'. *Sexualities, 21,* 743–746. https://doi.org/10.1177/1363460716684511.

Church, S., Henderson, M., Barnard, M., & Hart, G. (2001). Violence by clients towards female prostitutes in different work settings: Questionnaire survey. *British Medical Journal, 322,* 524–525. https://doi.org/10.1136/bmj.322.7285.524.

Comte, J. (2014). Decriminalization of sex work: Feminist discourses. *Sexuality and Culture, 18,* 196–217. https://doi.org/10.1007/s12119-013-9174-5.

Cunningham, S., Sanders, T., Platt, L., Grenfell, P., & Macioti, P. G. (2018). Sex work and occupational homicide: Analysis of a U.K. murder database. *Homicide Studies, 22,* 321–338. https://doi.org/10.1177/1088767918754306.

Dalla, R. L., Xia, Y., & Kennedy, H. (2003). "You just give them what they want pray they don't kill you": Street-level sex workers' reports of victimization, personal resources, and coping strategies. *Violence Against Women, 9,* 1367–1394. https://doi.org/10.1177/1077801203255679.

DeHart, D., Lynch, S., Belknap, J., Dass-Brailsford, P., & Green, B. (2014). Life history models of female offending: The roles of serious mental illness and trauma in women's pathways to jail. *Psychology of Women Quarterly, 38,* 138–151. https://doi.org/10.1177/0361684313494357.

Egger, S. (2002). *The killers among us: An examination of serial murder and its investigation* (2nd ed.). Upper Saddle River, NJ: Prentice Hall.

El-Bassel, N., Simoni, J. M., Cooper, D. K., Gilbert, L., & Schilling, R. F. (2001a). Sex trading and psychological distress among women on methadone. *Psychology of Addictive Behaviors, 15,* 177–184. https://doi.org/10.1037//0893-164X.15.3.177.

El-Bassel, N., Witte, S. S., Wada, T., Gilbert, L., & Wallace, J. (2001b). Correlates of partner violence among female street-based sex workers: Substance abuse, history of childhood abuse, and HIV risks. *AIDS Patient Care and STDs, 15,* 41–51. https://doi.org/10.1089/108729101460092.

Eller, L., & Mahat, G. (2003). Psychological factors in Nepali former commercial sex workers with HIV. *Journal of Nursing Scholarship, 35,* 53–60. https://doi.org/10.1111/j.1547-5069.2003.00053.x.

Farley, M., & Barkan, H. (1998). Prostitution, violence, and posttraumatic stress disorder. *Women and Health, 27,* 37–49. https://doi.org/10.1300/J013v27n03_03.

Farley, M., Lynne, J., & Cotton, A. J. (2005). Prostitution in Vancouver: Violence and the colonization of First Nations women. *Transcultural Psychiatry, 42,* 242–271. https://doi.org/10.1177/1363461505052667.

Farley, M., Cotton, A., Lynne, J., Zumbeck, S., Spiwak, F., Reyes, M. E., … Sezgin, U. (2003). Prostitution and trafficking in nine countries: An update on violence and posttraumatic stress disorder. *Journal of Trauma Practice*, *2*(3/4), 33–74. https://doi.org/10.1300/j189v02n03_03.

Folkes, I. (2013, August 26). Zurich introduces 'drive-in' sex. *BBC News*. Retrieved from https://www.bbc.com/news/world-europe-23839358.

Gilchrist, G., Gruer, L., & Atkinson, J. (2005). Comparison of drug use and psychiatric morbidity between prostitute and non-prostitute female drug users in Glasgow, Scotland. *Addictive Behaviors, 30,* 1019–1023. https://doi.org/10.1016/j.addbeh.2004.09.003.

Goffman, E. (1963). *Stigma: Notes on the management of spoiled identity*. Englewood Cliffs, NJ: Prentice-Hall.

Grandey, A. A. (2000). Emotion regulation in the workplace: A new way to conceptualize emotional labor. *Journal of Occupational Health Psychology, 5,* 95–110. https://doi.org/10.1037//1076-8998.5.1.95.

Gross, J. J. (1998). The emerging field of emotion regulation: An integrative review. *Review of General Psychology, 2,* 271–299. https://doi.org/10.1037/1089-2680.2.3.271.

Hammond, N. (2015). Men who pay for sex and the sex work movement? Client responses to stigma and increased regulation of commercial sex policy. *Social Policy & Society, 14,* 93–102. https://doi.org/10.1017/s1474746414000360.

Hammond, N., & Kingston, S. (2014). Experiencing stigma as sex work researchers in professional and personal lives. *Sexualities, 17,* 329–347. https://doi.org/10.1177/1363460713516333.

Harrell, E. (2011). *Workplace Violence, 1993–2009*. Report No. NCJ 233231. Retrieved from U.S. Department of Justice http://www.bjs.gov/content/pub/pdf/wv09.pdf.

Hochschild, A. R. (1983). *The managed heart: Commercialization of human feeling*. Berkeley: University of California Press.

Hong, Y., Li, X., Fang, X., & Zhao, R. (2007). Correlates of suicidal ideation and attempt among female sex workers in China. *Health Care for Women International, 28,* 490–505. https://doi.org/10.1080/07399330701226529.

Hong, Y., Fang, X., Li, X., Liu, Y., Li, M., & Tai-Seale, T. (2010). Self-perceived stigma, depressive symptoms and suicidal behaviors among female sex workers in China. *Journal of Transcultural Nursing, 21,* 29–34. https://doi.org/10.1177/1043659609349063.

Hughes, E. C. (1951). Work and the self. In J. H. Rohrer & M. Sherif (Eds.), *Social psychology at the crossroads* (pp. 313–323). New York: Harper & Brothers.

Hughes, E. C. (1958). *Men and their work.* Glencoe, IL: Free Press.

Ingram, R. E., & Luxton, D. D. (2005). Vulnerability-stress models. In B. L. Hankin & J. R. Z. Abela (Eds.), *Development of psychopathology: A vulnerability-stress perspective* (pp. 32–46). Thousand Oaks, CA: Sage.

Irvine, J. M. (2015). The other sex work: Stigma in sexuality research. *Social Currents, 2,* 116–125. https://doi.org/10.1177/2329496515579762.

Jonsson, S., & Jakobsson, N. (2017). Is buying sex morally wrong? Comparing attitudes toward prostitution using individual-level data across eight Western European countries. *Women's Studies International Forum, 61,* 58–69. https://doi.org/10.1016/j.wsif.2016.12.007.

Khantzian, E. J. (1997). The self-medication hypothesis of substance use disorders: A reconsideration and recent applications. *Harvard Review of Psychiatry, 4,* 231–244. https://doi.org/10.3109/10673229709030550.

Koken, J. A. (2012). Independent female escort's strategies for coping with sex work related stigma. *Sexuality and Culture, 16,* 209–229. https://doi.org/10.1007/s12119-011-9120-3.

Kramer, L. A. (2003). Emotional experiences of performing prostitution. *Journal of Trauma Practice, 2,* 187–197. https://doi.org/10.1300/j189v02n03_10.

Kraus, J. F. (1987). Homicide while at work: Persons, industries, and occupations at high risk. *American Journal of Public Health, 77,* 1285–1289.

Kreiner, G. E., Ashforth, B. E., & Sluss, D. M. (2006). Identity dynamics in occupational dirty work: Integrating social identity and system justification perspectives. *Organization Science, 17,* 619–636. https://doi.org/10.1287/orsc.1060.0208.

Krumrei-Mancuso, E. J. (2017). Sex work and mental health: A study of women in the Netherlands. *Archives of Sexual Behavior, 46,* 1843–1856. https://doi.org/10.1007/s10508-016-0785-4.

Lazarus, R. S. (1966). *Psychological stress and the coping process.* New York: McGraw-Hill.

Lazarus, R. S. (1993). From psychological stress to the emotions: A history of changing outlooks. *Annual Review of Psychology, 44,* 1–21. https://doi.org/10.1146/annurev.ps.44.020193.000245.

Matsueda, R. L., Gartner, R., Piliavan, I., & Polakowski, M. (1992). The prestige of criminal and conventional occupations: A subcultural model of criminal activity. *American Sociological Review, 57,* 752–770. https://doi.org/10.2307/2096121.

Miller, J., & Schwartz, M. D. (1995). Rape myths and violence against street prostitutes. *Deviant Behavior, 16,* 1–23. https://doi.org/10.1080/01639625.1995.9967984.

Molitor, F., Ruiz, J. D., Klausner, J. D., & McFarland, W. (2000). History of forced sex in association with drug use and sexual HIV risk behaviors, infection with STDs, and diagnostic medical care: Results from the Young Women Survey. *Journal of Interpersonal Violence, 15,* 262–278. https://doi.org/10.1177/088626000015003003.

Monto, M. A. (2010). Prostitutes' customers: Motives in misconceptions. In R. Weitzer (Ed.), *Sex for sale: Prostitution, pornography, and the sex industry* (2nd ed., pp. 233–254). New York: Routledge.

Neal, M. (2018). Dirty customers: Stigma and identity among sex tourists. *Journal of Consumer Culture, 18,* 131–148. https://doi.org/10.1177/1469540516648373.

Nixon, K., Tutty, L., Downe, P., Gorkoff, K., & Ursel, J. (2002). The everyday occurrence: Violence in the lives of girls exploited through prostitution. *Violence Against Women, 8,* 1016–1043. https://doi.org/10.1177/107780120200800902.

O'Doherty, T. (2011). Victimization in Off-street sex industry work. *Violence Against Women, 17,* 944–963. https://doi.org/10.1177/1077801211412917.

Odinokova, V., Rusakova, M., Urada, L. A., Silverman, J. G., & Raj, A. (2014). Police sexual coercion and its association with risky sex work and substance use behaviors among female sex workers in St. Petersburg and Orenburg, Russia. *International Journal of Drug Policy, 25,* 96–104. https://doi.org/10.1016/j.drugpo.2013.06.008.

Perdue, T. R., Williamson, C., Ventura, L. A., Hairston, T. R., Osborne, L. T., Laux, J. M., … Nathan, V. M. (2012). Offenders who are mothers with and without experience in prostitution: Differences in historical trauma, current stressors, and physical and mental health differences. *Women's Health Issues, 22,* e195–e200. https://doi.org/10.1016/j.whi.2011.08.01.

Phillips, R., Benoit, C., Hallgrimsdottir, H., & Vallance, K. (2012). Courtesy stigma: A hidden health concern to front-line service providers to sex workers. *Sociology of Health & Illness, 34,* 681–696. https://doi.org/10.1111/j.1467-9566.2011.01410.x.

Platt, L., Grenfell, P., Meiksin, R., Elmes, J., Sherman, S. G., Sanders, T., Mwangi, P., & Crago, A. L. (2018). Associations between sex work laws and sex workers' health: A systematic review and meta-analysis of quantitative and qualitative studies. *PLoS Medicine, 15*(12), e1002680. https://doi.org/10.1371/journal.pmed.1002680.

Popoola, B. I. (2013). Occupational hazards and coping strategies of sex workers in southwestern Nigeria. *Health Care for Women International, 34,* 139–149. https://doi.org/10.1080/07399332.2011.646366.

Potterat, J. J., Phillips, L., Rothenberg, R. B., & Darrow, W. (1985). On becoming a prostitute: An exploratory case-comparison study. *Journal of Sex Research, 21,* 329–335. https://doi.org/10.1080/00224498509551271.

Potterat, J. J., Brewer, D., Muth, S. Q., Rothenberg, R. B., Woodhouse, D. E., Muth, J. B., et al. (2004). Mortality in a long-term open cohort of prostitute women. *American Journal of Epidemiology, 159,* 778–785. https://doi.org/10.1093/aje/kwh110.

Quinet, K. (2011). Prostitutes as victims of serial homicide: Trends and case characteristics, 1970–2009. *Homicide Studies, 15,* 74–100.

Rael, C. T. (2015). Perceptions of sex work-related stigma in female sex workers from the Dominican Republic: Implications for HIV interventions. *Sexuality and Culture, 19,* 674–684. https://doi.org/10.1007/s12119-015-9284-3.

Rayson, J., & Alba, B. (2019). Experiences of stigma and discrimination as predictors of mental health help-seeking among sex workers. *Sexual and Relationship Therapy, 34,* 277–289. https://doi.org/10.1080/14681994.2019.1628488.

Rodriguez, E. M., Fuentes, P., Ramos-Lira, L., Gutierrez, R., & Ruiz, E. (2014). Violencia en el entorno laboral del trabajo sexual y consumo de sustancias en mujeres mexicanas [Violence in the work environment of sex work and substance use in a group of Mexican women]. *Salud Mental, 37,* 355–360. https://doi.org/10.17711/sm.0185-3325.2014.041.

Rössler, W. W., Koch, U. U., Lauber, C. C., Hass, A. K., Altwegg, M. M., Ajdacic-Gross, V. V., et al. (2010). The mental health of female sex workers. *Acta Psychiatrica Scandinavica, 122,* 143–152. https://doi.org/10.1111/j.1600-0447.2009.01533.x.

Roxburgh, A., Degenhardt, L., & Copeland, J. (2006). Posttraumatic stress disorder among female street-based sex workers in the greater Sydney area, Australia. *BMC Psychiatry, 6*(24). https://doi.org/10.1186/1471-244x-6-24.

Salfati, C. G., James, A. R., & Ferguson, L. (2008). Prostitute homicides: A descriptive study. *Journal of Interpersonal Violence, 23,* 505–543. https://doi.org/10.1177/0886260507312946.

Sanders, T. (2005). "It's just acting": Sex workers' strategies for capitalizing on sexuality. *Gender, Work and Organization, 12,* 319–342. https://doi.org/10.1111/j.1468-0432.2005.00276.x.

Sanders, T. (2018). Unpacking the process of destigmatization of sex work/ers: Response to Weitzer 'Resistance to sex work stigma'. *Sexualities, 21,* 736–739. https://doi.org/10.1177/1363460716677731.

Sanders, T., & Campbell, R. (2007). Designing out vulnerability, building in respect: Violence, safety, and sex work policy. *British Journal of Sociology, 58,* 1–19. https://doi.org/10.1111/j.1468-4446.2007.00136.x.

Sanders, T., Connelly, L., & King, L. J. (2016). On our own terms: The working conditions of internet sex workers in the UK. *Sociological Research Online, 21*(4). https://doi.org/10.5153/sro.4152.

Sanders, T., Scoular, J., Campbell, R., Pitcher, J., & Cunningham, S. (2018). *Internet sex work: Beyond the gaze*. London: Palgrave Macmillan.
Scambler, G., & Paoli, F. (2008). Health work, female sex workers and HIV/AIDS: Global and local dimensions of stigma and deviance as barriers to effective interventions. *Social Science and Medicine, 66,* 1848–1862. https://doi.org/10.1016/j.socscimed.2008.01.002.
Scutt, J. A. (1994). Judicial vision: Rape, prostitution, and the 'chaste woman'. *Women's Studies International Journal, 17,* 345–356. https://doi.org/10.1016/S0277-5395(05)80042-1.
Seib, C., Dunne, M. P., Fischer, J., & Najman, J. M. (2012). Predicting job satisfaction of female sex workers in Queensland, Australia. *International Journal of Sexual Health, 24,* 99–111. https://doi.org/10.1080/19317611.2011.632073.
Shaver, F. M. (1994). The regulation of prostitution: Avoiding the morality traps. *Canadian Journal of Law and Society, 9,* 123–145. https://doi.org/10.1017/s0829320100003537.
Shaver, F. M. (2005). Sex work research: Methodological and ethical challenges. *Journal of Interpersonal Violence, 20,* 296–319. https://doi.org/10.1177/0886260504274340.
Smith, M. (1943). An empirical scale of prestige status of occupations. *American Sociological Review, 8,* 185–192. https://doi.org/10.2307/2085884.
Stuewig, J., Tangney, J. P., Kendall, S., Folk, J. B., Meyer, C. R., & Dearing, R. L. (2015). Children's proneness to shame and guilt predict risky and illegal behaviors in young adulthood. *Child Psychiatry and Human Development, 46*(2), 217–227. https://doi.org/10.1007/s10578-014-0467-1, https://doiorg.lib.pepperdine.edu/.
Suresh, G., Furr, L., & Srikrishnan, A. (2009). An assessment of the mental health of street-based sex workers in Chennai, India. *Journal of Contemporary Criminal Justice, 25*(2), 186–201. https://doi.org/10.4135/9788132114109.n16.
Surratt, H. L., Inciardi, J. A., Kurtz, S. P., & Kiley, M. C. (2004). Sex work and drug use in a subculture of violence. *Crime & Delinquency, 50,* 43–59. https://doi.org/10.1177/0011128703258875.
Thompson, S. E. (2000). Prostitution—A choice ignored. *Women's Rights Law Reporter, 21,* 217–247.
Urada, L. A., Strathdee, S. A., Morisky, D. E., Schilling, R. F., Simbulan, N. P., Estacio, L. R., Jr., & Raj, A. (2014). Sex work and its associations with alcohol and methamphetamine use among female bar and Spa workers in the Philippines. *Asia-Pacific Journal of Public Health, 26,* 138–146. https://doi.org/10.1177/1010539512471969.
van Nunen, K., Leuridan, E., Van Hal, G., Van Damme, P., & Decorte, T. (2014). Legal and illegal drug use among female sex workers in bar and club prostitution in Belgium: A qualitative and quantitative study. *Drugs: Education, Prevention, and Policy, 21,* 56–64. https://doi.org/10.3109/09687637.2013.806432.
Vanwesenbeeck, I. (2001). Another decade of social scientific work on sex work: A review of research 1990–2000. *Annual Review of Sex Research, 12,* 242–287.
Vanwesenbeeck, I., de Graaf, R., van Zessen G., Straver, C., & Visser, J. (1993). Risky life, risky business: AIDS risk of female prostitutes in the context of early abuse and well-being. *Gedrag & Gezondheid, 21,* 219-26.
Ward, H., Day, S., & Weber, J. (1999). Risky business: Health and safety in the sex industry over a 9 year period. *Sexually Transmitted Infections, 75,* 340–343. https://doi.org/10.1136/sti.75.5.340.
Weitzer, R. (2007). Prostitution: Facts and fictions. *Contexts, 6*(4), 28–33. https://doi.org/10.1525/ctx.2007.6.4.28.
Weitzer, R. (2009). Sociology of sex work. *Annual Review of Sociology, 35,* 213–234. https://doi.org/10.1146/annurev-soc-070308-120025.
Weitzer, R. (2010). Sex work: Paradigms and policies. In R. Weitzer (Ed.), *Sex for sale: Prostitution, pornography, and the sex industry* (pp. 1–43). New York: Routledge.
Weitzer, R. (2012). *Legalizing prostitution: From illicit vice to lawful business*. New York: New York University Press.
Weitzer, R. (2018). Resistance to sex worker stigma. *Sexualities, 21,* 717–729. https://doi.org/10.1177/1363460716684509.

Whittaker, D., & Hart, G. (1996). Research note: Managing risks: The social organisation of indoor sex work. *Sociology of Health & Illness, 18,* 399–414. https://doi.org/10.1111/1467-9566.ep10934742.

YouGov (2016). Morality of accepting/paying money for sex [Data set]. Retrieved from https://d25d2506sfb94s.cloudfront.net/cumulus_uploads/document/xivicl1avj/tabs_OP_Prostitution_20160307.pdf.

Zehnder, M., Mutschler, J., Rössler, W., Rufer, M., & Rüsch, N. (2019). Stigma as a barrier to mental health service use among female sex workers in Switzerland. *Frontiers in Psychiatry, 10,* 32. https://doi.org/10.3389/fpsyt.2019.00032.

Zhang, C., Li, X., Hong, Y., Su, S., & Zhou, Y. (2014). Relationship between female sex workers and gatekeeper: The impact on female sex worker's mental health in China. *Psychology, Health & Medicine, 19,* 656–666. https://doi.org/10.1080/13548506.2013.869612.

Chapter 4
Selling Sex and Mental Health Concerns

Whether selling sex is associated with mental health concerns is central to sociopolitical debates about selling sex, including whether selling sex should be legal and how best to identify and support the needs of women who sell sex. There tends to be a social perception that selling sex is associated with mental health problems, but is this true or a myth? Does it depend on which mental health characteristics are considered? Does it change based on the setting or context of selling sex? If links can be established, can we conclude anything about causality? Does selling sex cause mental health concerns? Are those with mental health problems more likely to be drawn to selling sex? This chapter explores when, how, and to what extent mental health symptoms are associated with selling sex. We start by considering studies that have examined general or combined indicators of mental health, and then explore findings per mental health condition, including posttraumatic stress disorder, anxiety, depression, suicidality, dissociative disorders, somatic symptom disorder, personality disorders, and psychotic disorders. The literature indicates that certain themes relate to the prevalence of many mental health concerns, such as the context in which women sell sex (on the street vs. indoors), whether or not the women use or abuse drugs, and the extent to which they are victims of violence and abuse. Given this, we will explore these factors in relation to each relevant mental health issue.

Throughout this chapter, we compare the prevalence of specific mental health concerns among women who sell sex to the prevalence of these concerns among women who do not sell sex, such as women in a specific reference group or in the general population. As noted in Chap. 2, the general population is typically not an ideal comparison group, since it doesn't account for potentially unique features of samples of women who sell sex, such as geography, race, socioeconomic status, substance use, or history of violence and abuse. This concern is particularly relevant to this chapter on mental health, given the general finding that there are disparate rates of mental health diagnoses between individuals of different races and social classes (e.g., Coleman et al., 2016; Winstead & Sanchez, 2016). Nevertheless, we include general population data in our tables as a very imprecise reference point in

E. Krumrei Mancuso and B. E. Postlethwaite, *Women Who Sell Sex*,
https://doi.org/10.1007/978-3-030-47027-2_4

the absence of better comparison groups in the literature. We present study level and comparison data in tabular format when there are sufficient data to do so. To keep this review at a manageable length, the studies cited are intended to be illustrative rather than comprehensive in nature. Further, given the large number of studies that have been conducted on alcohol and substance abuse as a mental health outcome among women who sell sex, we will devote a separate chapter to this topic (Chap. 5).

General Mental Health Status and Other Indicators of Wellbeing

This chapter will review a great deal of research on specific mental health conditions among women who sell sex. First, we will review a number of studies examining mental health indexes of global measures of wellbeing. Some of this research has found no links between selling sex and poorer mental health. For example, an Australian study comparing women[1] selling sex to an age-matched sample of women from the general population found no differences in scores on a measure of common mental health problems, including depression, anxiety, somatic symptoms, and social withdrawal (Romans, Potter, Martin, & Herbison, 2001).

However, others have found links between selling sex and increased mental health concerns. De Schampheleire (1990) compared scores on the Minnesota Multiphasic Personality Inventory (MMPI) between women selling sex in Belgium and similar-aged women working for a Belgian airline. Compared to those working for the airline, women selling sex experienced higher levels of a number of mental health concerns, including hypochondriasis (now known as illness anxiety disorder), psychopathic deviance, paranoia, psychasthenia, schizophrenia, and hypomania. A similar trend was observed among women in New York receiving methadone maintenance treatment (El-Bassel, Simoni, Cooper, Gilbert, & Schilling, 2001). Those who had traded sex for money or drugs in the previous year scored higher than those who had not traded sex in the previous year on the General Severity Index of the Brief Symptom Inventory, a measure assessing a full range of mental health symptoms. Some research suggest that mental health status among women who sell sex is associated specifically with their levels of satisfaction with selling sex. A study of women selling sex in Australia indicated that better general mental health, defined as not having symptoms of depression or anxiety, was predictive of being more satisfied with selling sex (Seib, Dunne, Fischer, & Najman, 2012). This indicates that women who have symptoms of depression and anxiety are less likely to be happy with selling sex, however, it is unclear whether the experience of depression and anxiety results in dissatisfaction with selling sex and/or whether selling sex despite one's dissatisfaction with doing so is responsible for symptoms of anxiety and depression. Although

[1] The age range started at 16 years, with a mean age of 29 years. This is the same sample reported on by Potter, Martins, and Roman (1999).

causality between selling sex and mental health concerns is difficult to establish, longitudinal research is able to speak to directionality. For example, a study conducted among women receiving opioid agonist treatment who were assessed at seven time points, suggested there was an association in the direction of depression and anxiety resulting in women in this sample being more likely to sell sex in the future, given that symptoms of anxiety and depression were predictive of selling sex at future assessment points, even when controlling baseline levels of selling sex (Marchand et al., 2012).

With regard to global levels of wellbeing, research has indicated that women who sell sex may experience less satisfaction in life. An Australian study found that women selling sex were significantly less likely than women in other occupations to be satisfied with their lives overall (76 vs. 95%), their health (61 vs. 88%), their employment conditions (36 vs. 87%), their financial situations (49 vs. 71%), the homes in which they lived (58 vs. 89%), the neighborhoods in which they lived (72 vs. 92%), how safe they felt (61 vs. 94%), and the extent to which they felt a part of their local communities (39 vs. 73%; Bilardi et al., 2011).

The context in which women sell sex is a factor that may contribute to differences in whether women who sell sex do or do not experience increased risk of mental health concerns. This is illustrated by the work of Romans and colleagues (2001) who did not find differences in mental health indices between women selling sex and age-matched comparison women from the general population, but found differences among women selling sex. Specifically, those who worked in massage parlors and those who worked privately with regular customers fared better in terms of mental health than those who worked in other settings, including on the street, for an escort agency, or working privately through advertising. Along these lines, Exner, Wylie, Leura, and Parrill (1977) studied MMPI scores for women based on the venue where they sold sex, including call girls, those working in establishments (brothels, massage parlors, etc.), housewives, and those selling sex on the street. A comparison group of women was used for each group of women selling sex, that was matched on the basis of age, marital status, education, and socioeconomic status. Differences in mental health indices were much starker for some groups compared to others. The call girls and those working in indoor establishments scored similarly to their counterparts who did not sell sex, differing only on one variable each in relation to the comparison group (hypomania and hysteria, respectively). However, those who sold sex on the street scored higher than both their control group and the call girls in hysteria, psychopathic deviance, and social introversion. Women who sold sex on the street to support substance abuse or gambling displayed the worst outcomes, scoring higher than the control group and the other groups of women selling sex for many measures of psychopathology, including hypochondriasis (now known as illness anxiety disorder), depression, hysteria, psychopathic deviance, psychasthenia, schizophrenia, hypomania, and social introversion.

Research has indicated that age may also be a relevant factor in the link between selling sex and mental health indexes. Among a sample of women selling sex in Belgium, those 30 years or older scored higher on a number of MMPI scales than their younger counterparts under age 30, including psychasthenia, schizophrenia, hypomania, and social introversion (De Schampheleire, 1990). De Schampheleire did not hypothesize an explanation for this finding (his work was published posthumously after being prepared by an American psychologist). Age may be correlated with number of years spent selling sex, and hypotheses could be formed about increased distress over time. However, this finding may also be an artifact of general age-of-onset trends observed in large-scale epidemiological studies. For example, average age of onset of mood disorders is 29–43 years (interquartile range 35–40; Kessler et al., 2007). Thus, we might expect to see higher rates of mental health concerns for those over versus under 30 years, regardless of engagement in commercial sex. Next, this chapter explores a number of the themes raised in this section in more detail with regard to individual indicators of mental health.

Posttraumatic Stress Disorder

Posttraumatic stress disorder (PTSD) is one of the most commonly studied mental health concerns among women who sell sex. It involves symptoms in response to at least one major, distressing event from the past, including real or threatened injury or death to oneself or another person. Common symptoms include re-experiencing the traumatic event (e.g., flashbacks), emotional numbness, avoiding things that remind one of the event, and physical hyperarousal. It has been estimated that approximately one third of the general population will be exposed to a severe trauma during their lifetime, however, only a minority (10–20%) of those who experience trauma develop PTSD (Brunello et al., 2001). Data from the United States suggests that PTSD is twice as common among women as men, with half of women's cases being associated with sexual assault (Brunello et al., 2001).

Table 4.1 demonstrates from a sampling of studies that the prevalence of PTSD among women who sell sex tends to be higher than among women in the general population. Studies making use of matched control groups also indicate that those with a history of selling sex experience higher levels of PTSD than similar comparison individuals (e.g., Choi, Klein, Shin, & Lee, 2009; Jung, Song, Chong, Seo, & Chae, 2008; Perdue et al., 2012), with some exceptions where no differences were observed (e.g., DeHart, Lynch, Belknap, Dass-Brailsford, & Green, 2014). It is important to note that Table 4.1 demonstrates that PTSD prevalence among women who sell sex differs widely across studies, ranging from 8% among a sample of women selling sex in Malawi (MacLean et al., 2018) to 66% among a sample of women selling sex in Turkey (Farley et al., 2003). Some of this variance is likely due to methodological factors. For example, studies use different clinical tools and diagnostic criteria for determining levels of PTSD. In addition, prevalence is reported for different time frames ranging from current (e.g., past month, past year) to lifetime. In several studies, the time frame for PTSD is either unclear or unspecified. All of these methodological factors can make comparison between studies problematic. Next, we will explore some additional themes that may help explain the difference in PTSD prevalence

Table 4.1 Prevalence of PTSD among women selling sex and comparison samples

Study	Country	Venue	Sample size	Sexual violence history		PTSD prevalence	Prevalence time frame
				As a child	While selling sex		
MacLean et al. (2018)	Malawi	Indoor	200	Not specified	Not specified	8%	Past month
Rössler et al. (2010)	Switzerland	Mixed	193	Not specified	20%	13% 21%	Past year Lifetime
Cwikel et al. (2003)	Israel	Indoors	55	33%	30%	17%	Past month
Iaisuklang & Ali (2018)	India	Mixed	100	Not specified	Not specified	21%	Current
Daalder et al. (2013)	The Netherlands	Indoors	123[a]	42%	Not specified	23%	Past month
Roxburgh et al. (2006)	Australia	Outdoors	72	75%	>40%	31% 47%	Current Lifetime
Coetzee et al. (2018)	South Africa	Not specified	508	Not specified	Not specified	38%	Current
Valera et al. (2000)	USA	Outdoors	42	44%	74%	41%	Not specified
Farley et al. (2003)	Mexico	Mixed	123	54%	46%	54%	Not specified
Suresh et al. (2009)	India	Outdoors	57	Not specified	Not specified[b]	56%	Past month
Farley et al. (2003)	Turkey	Unclear	50[c]	34%	50%	66%	Not specified

(continued)

Table 4.1 (continued)

Study	Country	Venue	Sample size	Sexual violence history		PTSD prevalence	Prevalence time frame
				As a child	While selling sex		
Comparison population: U.S. adult females (2001–2003)							
Harvard Medical School (2007a, b)[d]	USA		5692[e]			5% 10%	Past year Lifetime
Comparison sample: U.S. adult female offenders							
DeHart et al. (2014)	USA		115	48%		51%	Lifetime

Notes Sexual Violence History: As a child = % of sample reporting sexual assault/molestation as a minor; While selling Sex: % of sample reporting sexual violence while selling sex

[a]Daalder et al. (2013) included participants as young as 17 years

[b] Suresh et al. (2009) reported 67% of their sample experienced serious violence while working, but did not specify a percentage for sexual violence, specifically

[c]Farley et al. (2003) included participants as young as 16 years

[d]Data from the National Comorbidity Survey Replication

[e]Sample size includes men. Sample size was not specified per gender, although women are expected to make up roughly half of this nationally representative sample

between women who sell sex and women in the general population, as well as the variance in PTSD prevalence among different samples of women who sell sex.

Lifetime Abuse and Violence as Predictors of PTSD

Experiences prior to, and outside of the context of selling sex likely contribute to PTSD among women who sell sex. Childhood sexual abuse (Choi et al., 2009; Valera, Sawyer, & Schiraldi, 2000), childhood physical abuse (Valera et al., 2000), childhood emotional abuse (Daalder, Bogaerts, & Bijleveld, 2013), childhood neglect (Roxburgh, Degenhardt, & Copeland, 2006), and adult sexual assault (Roxburgh et al., 2006) have all been associated with PTSD among women who sell sex. As detailed in Chaps. 2 and 3, women who sell sex tend to have experienced more abuse and violence in both childhood and adulthood than those in the general population, offering one explanation for the higher prevalence of PTSD among those who sell sex.

Experiences While Selling Sex as Predictors of PTSD

A number of studies have indicated more time spent selling sex is associated with a higher likelihood of developing PTSD. For example, a study of women[2] selling sex indoors in the Netherlands indicated that the mean number of working hours was significantly higher for women with PTSD than for women without PTSD (Daalder et al., 2013). Along similar lines, a Korean study of women in shelters with a history of selling sex indicated that a longer duration of selling sex was associated with a greater severity of PTSD symptoms (Jung et al., 2008). It is possible that past trauma histories contribute to women choosing to sell sex and spending more time selling sex, making past trauma history the explanatory variable between selling sex to a greater extent and the experience of PTSD. However, there is more research support for the idea that women are exposed to experiences while selling sex that increase their likelihood of developing or progressing in PTSD symptoms. This is consistent with the description in the Diagnostic and Statistical Manual of Mental Disorders (DSM-5), that PTSD symptoms become more severe and persistent on the basis of longer exposure to trauma. There is empirical evidence that experiencing violence while selling sex is associated with PTSD (Cwikel, Ilan, & Chudakov, 2003[3]; Sanders, 2004; Suresh,

[2]The age range of this sample started at 17 years, with an average age of 33.5 years.

[3]This is the same sample as described by Chudakov, Ilan, Belmaker, and Cwikel (2002). We indicated in Chapter 1 that we systematically excluded studies of human trafficking victims, therefore, we should note that 82% of this sample had arrived into Israel illegally and could be considered trafficked. We retained this study because less than 4% of the sample indicated they were trafficked

Furr, & Srikrishnan, 2009). Violence while selling sex has been reported frequently, but the levels differ dramatically based on a number of factors, including the settings in which women work. For example, a study of women selling sex in the UK in saunas, brothels, from home, or as escorts, and to a lesser extent in the street, found that 29% of the women reported having experienced violence while selling sex (Sanders, 2004), whereas a study of women from the same country exclusively selling sex in the street found that 75% of women reported experiencing violence while selling sex (Sanders, 2001). A study demonstrating how such differences in violence per setting are associated with levels of PTSD was conducted in Switzerland by Rössler and colleagues (2010), who used cluster analyses to identify four groups of women: (1) those who were native Swiss and worked outdoors, experiencing high levels of violence and rape, with 12% prevalence of PTSD; (2) those who were of various ethnicities and worked in brothels, salons, or cabarets, experiencing low levels of violence, with 6% PTSD; (3) those who were of mixed-European origin and worked in studios, experiencing low levels of violence, with 0% PTSD; and (4) those who were mainly non-European and worked in studios, experiencing the highest levels of violence, with 40% PTSD.

Other Risk and Resilience Factors for PTSD

It should be noted that experiencing trauma while selling sex does not always result in PTSD. For example, Roxburgh et al. (2006) found that rates of physical assault while selling sex were equally high for women with PTSD and without PTSD (77% in both groups). The fact that some women encounter violence in the course of selling sex without developing PTSD is consistent with the definition of PTSD as a *pathological* response to the experience of trauma. In the general population, 80–90% of people who go through a trauma will not develop PTSD (Brunello et al., 2001). Whether a person develops PTSD following a trauma will depend on a host of risk and resilience factors (Agaibi & Wilson, 2005). Resilience factors that may keep some women from developing PTSD include having access to healthy coping strategies, having social support, or joining a support group. Risk factors for PTSD that are more common among some samples of women who sell sex include having little or no social support after the traumatic experience, experiencing other mental health symptoms, engaging in substance abuse, and facing other sources of stress in addition to a traumatic experience. Furthermore, there is a cumulative effect of abuse and violence when it comes to developing PTSD, that is, more instances of violence from childhood through adulthood, and experiencing more types of violence (e.g., physical, sexual) are correlated with developing PTSD for women who sell sex (Farley et al., 2003; Roxburgh et al., 2006; Sanders, 2004).

---

against their will. Almost all women reported selling sex of their own volition, even though 17% of the sample indicated being sold against their wishes to a brothel owner.

The importance of risk and resilience factors is also demonstrated by Rössler et al.'s (2010) Swiss clusters, where both clusters 3 and 4 consisted of women working in studios, but cluster 3 with 0% PTSD consisted of women from European origin and cluster 4 with 40% PTSD consisted of women of mostly non-European origin. Those from non-European origin experienced higher levels of violence, and may have faced a number of additional PTSD risk factors related to being ethnic minorities, living far from their countries of origin, experiencing poorer social treatment and less social support, and perhaps having less education and financial resources. Thus, in evaluating the differences in PTSD experienced by women who sell sex, including in relation to comparison samples, it is important to consider the entire spectrum of risk and resilience factors.

Anxiety

Anxiety disorders are characterized by excessive worries, fears, or apprehensions surrounding real or imagined objects or situations. Anxiety can present in a variety of forms, such as longer-term generalized anxiety about many different things or discrete panic attacks that involve unexpected periods of intense fear with physiological hyperarousal. Table 4.2 displays the prevalence of anxiety among samples of women who sell sex. Many of the studies providing statistics on the prevalence of anxiety among women who sell sex have been conducted among women who use drugs, a factor we have highlighted in the table due to the fact that this can limit the generalizability of these results to other women. The table provides the prevalence of anxiety for women in the general population and women who use drugs but do not sell sex as reference points. The prevalence of anxiety among women selling sex ranged from 8% in a sample from India (Iaisuklang & Ali, 2018) to 60% in a sample from Scotland (Gilchrist, Gruer, & Atkinson, 2005). However, it should be noted that anxiety was measured differently across studies. Although most studies used validated measures to evaluate levels of anxiety on the basis of clinically significant cut-off scores, some research made use of a single item to assess self-reported anxiety (e.g., Burnette et al., 2008). Further, the type of anxiety assessed is not always specified in the literature. Thus, differences in measurement may contribute to the diversity in prevalence of anxiety reported across studies.

Some research comparing women who sell sex to those who do not, has found no differences between the two groups. For example, a study of drug using women in Scotland comparing those who had and had not sold sex found levels of anxiety to be equally high among both groups (Gilchrist et al., 2005). Compared to the general population, women who sell sex tend to display a higher prevalence of anxiety (see Table 4.2). Although, comparison studies show that rates of anxiety differ depending on the contexts and characteristics of women who sell sex (e.g., Rössler et al., 2010). A number of qualitative studies have explored the reasons that some women who sell sex experience anxiety. A common theme is that anxiety can be a response to social stigma (e.g., Koken, 2012). In addition, selling sex can result in a host of difficulties in interpersonal relationships, often related to dishonesty, distrust, jealousy, stigma, and

Table 4.2 Prevalence of anxiety among women selling sex and comparison samples

Study	Country	Venue	Sample size	Current drug users	Type of anxiety assessed	Anxiety prevalence (%)	Prevalence time frame
Iaisuklang & Ali (2018)	India	Mixed	100	12%	Generalized anxiety	8	Current
Burnette et al. (2008)	USA	Not specified	816	100%[a]	Sudden irrational fear[b]	29	Past year
Rössler et al. (2010)	Switzerland	Mixed	193	Not specified	Any anxiety disorder	34 34	Past year Lifetime
					Generalized anxiety	5 7	Past year Lifetime
Ranjbar et al. (2018)	Iran	Outdoor	48	Not specified	Any anxiety disorder	37	Current
Surratt et al. (2005)	USA	Outdoor	278	100%[c]	Generalized anxiety	37	Past week
Ghose et al. (2015)[d]	India	Indoor	100	Not specified	Generalized anxiety/panic	44	Current
Gilchrist et al. (2005)	Scotland	Not specified	176	100%	Generalized anxiety	60	Current
Comparison population: U.S. adult females (2001–2003)							
Harvard Medical School (2007a, b)[e]	USA		>2073[f]		Any anxiety disorder[g]	23 36	Past year Lifetime
Comparison population: U.S. adult females (2001–2003)							
Harvard Medical School (2007a, b)[e]	USA		>2073[f]		Generalized anxiety	3 7	Past year Lifetime
Comparison population: U.S. adult female substance users who have not sold sex							
Burnette et al. (2008)	USA		790	100%[a]	Sudden irrational fear[b]	20	Past year
Comparison sample: Scottish female drug users who have not sold sex							
Gilchrist et al. (2005)	Scotland		176	100%	Generalized anxiety	53	Current

[a] Burnette et al.'s (2008) participants had all entered substance abuse treatment
[b] Burnette et al. (2008) used a single-item to assess feeling suddenly frightened or nervous in a situation in which other people would not have been afraid or nervous
[c] All of Surratt et al.'s (2005) participants used heroin and/or crack cocaine 3 × per week during the last 30 days
[d] All of Ghose et al.'s (2015) participants were infected with HIV
[e] Data from the National Comorbidity Survey Replication
[f] A range was provided for the sample size (2073–3197), which includes men; sample size was not specified per gender, although women are expected to make up roughly half of this nationally representative sample
[g] Included any DSM-5 anxiety disorder including panic disorder, specific phobia, social phobia, generalized anxiety disorder, obsessive-compulsive disorder, and PTSD

pragmatic issues surrounding disclosing information about selling sex, all of which can contribute to anxiety (Bellhouse, Crebbin, Fairley, & Bilardi, 2015; Sanders, 2004; Tomura, 2009). That is, women often experience tension about maintaining secrecy about their involvement in commercial sex or feel anxious about when and how to disclose that they sell sex. A lesser examined topic is whether anxiety also stems from intrapersonal feelings of guilt or shame about selling sex. Finally, some women experience anxiety surrounding the possibility of encountering violence or abuse while selling sex (Sanders, 2004).

Depression

Major depressive disorder, or depression, is a mood disorder characterized by sadness and/or a loss of interest in activities. It can include feelings of hopelessness, a loss of energy, difficulty concentrating, and changes in appetite and sleep. Table 4.3 shows the prevalence of moderate to severe depression among women who sell sex with statistics for comparison groups. The prevalence of depression among women who sell sex varies considerably across studies, ranging from 8% in a sample from Malawi (MacLean et al., 2018) to nearly 87% in a sample of women who sold sex on the street in Alegría et al., (1994). In most of these studies, depression was measured on the basis of being clinically diagnosable, on the basis of being severe, or on the basis of the number of symptoms being high. Most studies used validated measures to evaluate depressive symptoms on the basis of clinically significant scores, however, at least some research made use of a single item to assess depression (e.g., Burnette et al., 2008).

In considering the literature as a whole, women who sell sex seem to experience a high prevalence of depression. To offer some comparisons, the prevalence of depression among women selling sex appears to be greater than what is seen in the general population, but is mostly lower than what is seen among women entering substance abuse treatment. A number of studies have made use of specific comparison samples, mostly indicating that women who sell sex are more likely to experience depression than those who do not. In a Korean study, women recruited from shelters who used to sell sex experienced more depression than two comparison groups of women, including those living in the communities surrounding the shelters and field workers at the shelters (Jung et al., 2008). Those who had sold sex also experienced more symptoms associated with depression, such as fatigue, frustration, and problems sleeping, in comparison to the two other groups. Similarly, several studies of predominantly drug-using women have noted that depression was higher among those who sold sex than those who did not (El-Bassel et al., 1997; Risser, Timpson, McCurdy, Ross, & Williams, 2006). However, some research has found no links (Burnette et al., 2008) or no differences in levels of clinical depression, despite higher levels of depressive thinking among those who have sold sex compared to those who have not (Gilchrist et al., 2005). Among offender samples in the United States, the results have also been mixed, with some studies showing that women who had ever sold sex were more

Table 4.3 Prevalence of depression among women selling sex and comparison samples

Study	Country	Venue	Sample size	Current drug users	Depression prevalence (%)	Depression prevalence time frame
MacLean et al. (2018)	Malawi	Indoor	200	Not specified	8	Past 2 weeks
Iaisuklang & Ali (2018)	India	Mixed	100	12%	9 25	Current Past
Chudakov et al. (2002)	Israel	Indoor	55	Not specified	19	Past week
Ortblad et al. (2019)	Uganda	Mixed	262 297 302	Not specified	21 28 32	Current
Patterson et al. (2019)	Mexico (Cd. Juarez)	Mixed	129	71%	23	Current
Rössler et al. (2010)	Switzerland	Mixed	193	Not specified	24 36	Past year Lifetime
Ghose et al. (2015)	India	Indoor	100[a]	Not specified	30	Current
Hong et al. (2010)	China	Indoor	310	Not specified	30	Current
Jana et al. (2017)	India	Indoor	400	Not specified	38	Current
Patterson et al. (2019)	Mexico (Tijuana)	Mixed	141	54%	42	Current
Alegría et al. (1994)	Puerto Rico	Indoor	52	47%[b]	45	Current
Akcali et al. (2017)	Turkey	Indoor	108	3%	48	Current
Abelson et al. (2019)	Cameroon	Mixed	2165	Not specified	50[c]	Current
Ross et al. (2003)	Turkey	Indoor	50	20%	50	Current
Surratt et al. (2005)	USA	Outdoor	278	100%[d]	53	Past 2 weeks
Lau et al. (2010)	Hong Kong	Indoor	293	40%	54	Past week
Roxburgh et al. (2006)	Australia	Outdoor	72	94%[e]	54	Current
Ross et al. (2003)	Canada	Outdoor	20	55%	60	Current

(continued)

Table 4.3 (continued)

Study	Country	Venue	Sample size	Current drug users	Depression prevalence (%)	Depression prevalence time frame
Carlson et al. (2017)	Mongolia	Mixed	Not specified	Not specified	60	Past week
Burnette et al. (2008)	USA	Not specified	816	100%[f]	62[g]	Past year
Coetzee et al. (2018)	South Africa	Mixed	508	Not specified	66	Past week
Gilchrist et al. (2005)	Scotland	Not specified	176	100%	70	Current
Rael & Davis (2017)	Dominican Republic	Mixed	349	Not specified	70	Past week
Alegría et al. (1994)	Puerto Rico	Outdoor	75	47%[b]	87	Current
Comparison population: U.S. adult females (2001–2003)						
Harvard Medical School (2007a, b)[h]	USA		9282[i]		9 20	Past year Lifetime
Comparison population: U.S. adult female substance users who have not sold sex						
Burnette et al. (2008)	USA		790	100%[f]	62[g]	Past year
Comparison population: Scottish female substance users who have not sold sex						
Gilchrist et al. (2005)	Scotland		89	100%	61	Current

Note Unless otherwise noted, depression prevalence refers to moderate to severe depressive symptoms or clinical depression/major depressive disorder
[a]All of Ghose et al.'s (2015) participants were infected with HIV
[b]For Alegría et al. (1994), Drug User % refers to injection drug users in the combined indoor/outdoor sample
[c]Represents any level of depression (mild to severe)
[d]All of Surratt et al.'s (2005) participants used heroin and/or crack cocaine 3 × per week during the last 30 days
[e]For Roxburgh et al. (2006), Drug User % refers to lifetime history of injection drug use rather than current drug use
[f]All of Burnette et al.'s (2008) participants had entered substance abuse treatment
[g]Burnette et al. (2008) used a single-item to assess feeling very sad or depressed for two weeks or more during the past year
[h]Data from the National Comorbidity Survey Replication
[i]Sample size includes men. Sample size was not specified per gender, although women are expected to make up roughly half of this nationally representative sample

likely to experience clinical depression (Perdue et al., 2012) and other studies showing no difference in depression among those who had and had not sold sex (DeHart et al., 2014). Next, we explore some themes that may relate to the prevalence of depression among women who sell sex.

The Phenomenological Experience of Selling Sex in Relation to Depression

Kramer (2003) quantitatively explored the phenomenological experience of selling sex among a sample of mostly incarcerated women in the United States, among whom 66% had sold sex predominantly in the street and 33% had sold sex predominantly indoors. She found that more women identified the act of selling sex as emotionally painful than emotionally pleasurable (76 vs. 13%). She asked women to list five words that described their feelings while selling sex, and found that 90% of the descriptors had negative valence, with the most predominant theme being sadness (sad, depressed, empty, hopeless, helpless, unhappy, powerless, distraught, upset, etc.). Thus, for some women, the act of selling sex, itself, is associated with symptoms of depression. Although we should note that there are exceptions to this. For example, Sanders, Connelly, and King (2016) explored how 240 internet escorts in the UK (82% of whom were women) described their jobs. They noted that a small percentage of escorts described their jobs using negative terms such as dehumanizing (15%) and exploitative (14%), but that six of the top seven job characteristics chosen to describe selling sex were positive in nature (flexible, fun, rewarding, skillful, sociable, and empowering).

Violence and Abuse as Predictors of Depression

As is true for PTSD, the experience of violence is associated with increased depression. This is the case for violence experienced while selling sex (Cwikel et al., 2003; Sanders, 2004), as well as violence in intimate relationships outside of selling sex (Sanders, 2004). This mirrors findings among women in the general population, where the experience of violence is associated with higher rates of depression (Ellsberg, Jansen, Heise, Watts, & García-Moreno, 2008).

The Nature of the Venue as a Predictor of Depression

The studies included in Table 4.3 suggest that the prevalence of depression is higher for women who sell sex outdoors compared to indoors in brothels, hotels, or apartments. This finding is not surprising given the notoriously harsh environment of selling sex on the street. A small number of studies have comparatively examined the relationship between work venues and depression. For example, among women selling sex in Puerto Rico, those working on the street were significantly more likely to experience high levels of depressive symptoms than those working in brothels (87 vs. 45%; Alegría et al., 1994). However, research has indicated that not all indoor locations are equivalent, with regard to their links to depression. For example, Rössler and colleagues (2010) found that Swiss women selling sex on the street had a higher rate of 1-year depression diagnoses (46%) than European women selling sex primarily indoors in brothels or salons (15%) or in studios (10%). However, depression was equally high among non-European women selling sex indoors in studios (47%) as it was among the Swiss women working on the street (46%).

A large study of women selling sex in China offers additional insight into the factors associated with work venues that may contribute to differing levels of depression (Zhang et al., 2014). This study found venues that generated lower monthly incomes were associated with higher levels of depression. Further, women who had closer relationships with their managers in terms of trust, communication, and support, had less depression and loneliness, and better hopefulness for the future, even when controlling demographic characteristics. However, when adding alcohol and drug use and partner violence as controls, a positive relationship with one's manager was no longer predictive of levels of depression, although it remained predictive of levels of loneliness and hopefulness. This highlights that the experience of violence and use of alcohol/drugs are more important predictors of depression than the relationship with venue managers.

Substance and Alcohol Use as Predictors of Depression

As noted, a factor that can contribute to depression among women who sell sex is substance and alcohol use (e.g., Zhang et al., 2014). Research in the general population has demonstrated high comorbidity of substance use and depression (e.g., Regier et al., 1990). Some women use substances to self-medicate in response to depression and other forms of distress. However, drug use, itself, can also cause neurobiological changes that increase the risk of developing depression or exacerbate existing depressive symptoms (Volkow, 2004). This is relevant, given that substance use is prevalent among many research samples of women who sell sex (see Table 4.3).

Suicidality

When considering mental health concerns surrounding suicidality, it is relevant to consider completed suicides, attempted suicides, and suicidal ideation or thoughts about carrying out suicide. Table 4.4 shows the prevalence of some suicidal ideation and suicide attempts among women selling sex and comparison groups. As with other mental health concerns, these variables range considerably across studies. Suicidal ideation ranges from approximately 9% in a sample from South Africa (Coetzee et al., 2018) to 74% in a sample from Australia (Roxburgh et al., 2006). Suicide attempts range from approximately 8% in a sample from China (Hong, Li, Fang, & Zhao, 2007) to 53% in a sample from Scotland (Gilchrist et al., 2005).

Most studies have found rates of suicidality to be considerably higher among women selling sex than among the general population. However, rates of suicide and suicidality may or may not be higher for women who sell sex than for more relevant comparison groups. For example, among a sample of drug using women in Scotland, those who had sold sex were more likely to have attempted suicide than those who had not sold sex (a staggering 53% versus 39%, respectively; Gilchrist et al., 2005). However, other research has suggested suicidality is not higher among women who sell sex than among other high-risk populations. For example, a study from rural China found relatively high levels of suicidal ideation and suicide attempts among women who sold sex (14% and 8% respectively), but the numbers were similar to those previously reported for adolescent girls in rural China (Hong, Li, Fang, & Zhao, 2007).

Factors contributing to increased suicidal ideation and attempts among women who sell sex include issues directly and indirectly related to selling sex as well as other psychological and life factors. In the context of selling sex, both age and reasons for starting to sell sex have been highlighted as relevant factors. Starting to sell selling sex as a juvenile is associated with higher risk of attempted suicide than starting to sell sex as an adult (31% versus 18%, respectively; Clarke, Clarke, Roe-Sepowitz, & Fey, 2012). In addition, research has indicated that women who report relationship failure or being deceived or forced as reasons for selling sex are more likely to experience suicidal ideation and suicide attempts than those who indicate their reasons for selling sex are financial needs or influence from peers (Hong et al., 2007).

As has been seen for other mental health concerns, differences also exist on the basis of work venue (highlighted in Table 4.4). Hong et al. (2007) found that women selling sex in hair salons were more likely to have had suicidal ideation and attempts than their counterparts selling sex in restaurants. Additionally, having a less positive relationships with venue managers in terms of trust, communication, and support has been associated with more suicidal intention and attempts (Zhang et al., 2014).

Many other variables have been linked to suicidality among women who sell sex, without much clarity about whether or how these findings are unique to women selling sex. In China, dissatisfaction with life, alcohol and drug use, experience of sexual coercion or partner violence, worry about not making enough money, and having a stable sexual partner have all been associated with higher risk of suicidal

Table 4.4 Prevalence of suicidal ideation and attempts among women selling sex and comparison samples

Study	Country	Venue	Sample size	Current drug users	Prevalence (%)	Prevalence time frame
Suicidal ideation						
Coetzee et al. (2018)	South Africa	Mixed	508	Not specified	9	Past year
Hong et al. (2007)	China	Indoor	454	Not specified	14	Past 6 month
Hong et al. (2010)	China	Indoor	310	Not specified	18	Past 6 month
Lau et al. (2010)	Hong Kong	Indoor	293	40%	38	Past 6 month
Cwikel et al. (2003)	Israel	Indoor	55	6%	41	Lifetime
Teixeira & Oliveira (2017)	Portugal	Outdoor	52	33%	46	Current
Roxburgh et al. (2006)	Australia	Outdoor	72	94%[a]	74	Lifetime
Suicide attempts						
Hong et al. (2007)	China	Indoor	454	Not specified	8	Past 6 month
Hong et al. (2010)	China	Indoor	310	Not specified	9	Past 6 month
Coetzee et al. (2018)	South Africa	Mixed	508	Not specified	10	Past year
Burnette et al. (2008)	USA	Not specified	816	100%[b]	14 41	Recent Lifetime
Clarke et al. (2012)	USA	Mixed	308	>39%	18	Lifetime
Cwikel et al. (2003)	Israel	Indoor	55	Not specified	19	Lifetime
Jung et al. (2013)	South Korea	Indoor	1083	Not specified	28	Past year
Suresh et al. (2009)	India	Outdoor	57	Not specified	~30	Lifetime
Roxburgh et al. (2006)	Australia	Outdoor	72	47%[a]	42	Lifetime

(continued)

Table 4.4 (continued)

Study	Country	Venue	Sample size	Current drug users	Prevalence (%)	Prevalence time frame
Teixeira & Oliveira (2017)	Portugal	Outdoor	52	33%	44	Lifetime
Gilchrist et al. (2005)	Scotland	Not specified	176	100%	53	Lifetime
Comparison population: U.S. adult females (2016), suicidal ideation & attempt						
Substance Abuse & Mental Health Services Administration (2017)[c]	USA		27,181	Ideation	4	Past year
				Attempts	1	
Comparison sample: U.S. adult females aged 18–54 (1990s), suicidal ideation & attempts						
Weissman et al. (1999)[d]	USA		7640[e]	Ideation Attempts	18 6	Lifetime
Comparison sample: U.S. adult female substance users who have not sold sex, suicide attempts						
Burnette et al. (2008)	USA		790[b]	Attempts	10 29	Recent Lifetime
Comparison sample: Scottish adult female drug users who have not sold sex, suicide attempts						
Gilchrist et al. (2005)	Scotland		89	Attempts	39	Lifetime

[a]For Roxburgh et al. (2006), Drug User % refers to lifetime history of injection drug use, rather than current drug users
[b]All of Burnette et al.'s (2008) participants had entered substance abuse treatment
[c]Data from the National Survey on Drug Use and Health (NSDUH) from the Substance Abuse and Mental Health Services Administration (SAMHSA), Tables 8.66B and 8.68B
[d]Data from the National Comorbidity Survey
[e]Sample size includes men. Sample size was not specified per gender, although women are expected to make up roughly half of this nationally representative sample

ideation or attempt among women who sell sex (Hong et al., 2007; Zhang et al., 2014). A stratified cluster random sampling of women selling sex throughout South Korea indicated that frequent alcohol consumption and having a sexually transmitted infection were both associated with suicide attempts (Jung, 2013). Many of these factors parallel findings in the general population, for example, alcohol or drug use disorders have widely been associated with increased risk of suicidal ideation and attempts (e.g., Borges & Loera, 2010).

Dissociative Disorders

There are a number of distinct dissociative disorders, including dissociative identity disorder, dissociative amnesia, and depersonalization/derealization disorder. These conditions are typically associated with past traumas, and the risk of dissociative disorders increase on the basis of the severity, frequency, and violence of the trauma experienced. They involve some form of amnesia or detachment from oneself, which can serve the function of mental escape from stressful, undesired situations. For example, amnesia might present in the form of forgetting particularly stressful commercial sex experiences; depersonalization, which involves a sense of disconnection from oneself, can present as a woman feeling robotic or like she is on autopilot while having sex with a customer, or even feeling like her body doesn't belong to her; identity confusion can involve uncertainty or conflict about one's sense of self related to selling sex; and in very rare cases, escaping into a role or alternate persona while selling sex could present as experiencing two or more distinct personality states.

The literature has highlighted that some women experience feelings of detachment or disconnection while selling sex (e.g., 11% of participants described by Kramer, 2003). However, research specifically examining dissociative disorders among women who sell sex is rare, and studies that have been conducted have made use of small samples. Table 4.5 shows the prevalence of dissociative disorders from two studies of women selling sex, as well as prevalence in the general population. Given the limited data available, these numbers should not be considered representative of the prevalence of dissociative disorders among women who sell sex. Further, the age range of the samples of women selling sex is unclear, therefore, minors may have been included in these studies.

In a small study, Ross, Anderson, Heber, and Norton (1990) compared the frequency of dissociative disorders among women selling sex, women who were exotic dancers, and women who had been diagnosed with multiple personality disorder (now known as dissociative identity disorder). Women selling sex displayed similar or lower frequencies of dissociative disorders than exotic dancers and lower frequencies of all forms of dissociative disorders than women diagnosed with multiple personality disorder.

Finally, not much is known about the outcomes of dissociative disorders for women who sell sex. There is some indication that it may be related to less adherence

Table 4.5 Limited data on prevalence of dissociative disorders among women selling sex and comparison samples

Study	Country	Venue	Sample size	Disorder prevalence (%)	Disorder type
Ross et al. (2003)[a]	Turkey	Indoor	50	20	Dissociative Amnesia
				18	Depersonalization
				18	Dissociative identity disorder
				4	Dissociative Fugue
				12	Dissociate disorder, not specified
Ross et al. (1990)[a]	Canada (Winnepeg)	Outdoor	20	35	Dissociative Amnesia
				15	Depersonalization
				5	Dissociative identity disorder
Comparison sample: adult females in Turkey, dissociative identity disorder (lifetime)					
Şar et al. (2007)	Turkey		628	7	Dissociative Amnesia
				1	Depersonalization
				1	Dissociative identity disorder
				0.2	Dissociative Fugue
				8	Dissociate disorder, not specified
Comparison sample: U.S. adult females, dissociative identity disorder (last year)					
Johnson et al. (2006)	USA		349	3	Dissociative Amnesia
				1	Depersonalization
				1	Dissociative identity disorder
				4	Dissociate disorder, not specified

[a]An age range was not provided by Ross et al. (1990) or Ross et al. (2003); it is unclear if minors were included in these samples

to prostitution-exiting programs. In a small study of women in the United States, dissociation stood out as a predictor of whether women completed a 90-day, residential prostitution-exiting program (Roe-Sepowitz, Hickle, & Cimino, 2012). Participation in the program was voluntary and the women who participated were offered a variety of support services including housing, employment or education assistance, and weekly counseling. Women with higher levels of dissociation when beginning the program were more likely to leave the program before completing it in comparison to women with lower levels of dissociation. Dissociation was the only symptom that was predictive of program completion, out of a range of mental health concerns, including anxiety, depression, irritability, intrusiveness, avoidance, and other trauma symptoms.

Somatic Symptom Disorder

Somatic Symptom Disorder is characterized by distress and abnormal thoughts, feelings, or behaviors in response to somatic symptoms, such as physical pain, numbness, tingling, dizziness, nausea, or other physical symptoms. Women in certain cultures may be more likely to report somatic symptoms over other mental health concerns, because medical problems are more socially accepted than mental problems (e.g., women selling sex in Nepal; Eller & Mahat, 2003).

A number of studies have indicated that women who sell sex are at increased risk for somatic symptom disorders compared to those who do not sell sex. In two studies from South Korea, women who had sold sex experienced significantly more somatic symptoms than a number of comparison groups, including an age and education matched control group and control women from the same community (Choi et al., 2009; Jung et al., 2008). Moreover, women who have sold sex for a longer period of time seem to have more somatic symptoms than those who are newer to commercial sex (Ulibarri et al., 2009).

In addition, an early study examining differences between women selling sex in different settings found that upper class call girls who worked with high paying customers scored lower on the MMPI scale of hysteria than women working in other settings, including brothels and street-based work (Exner, Wylie, Leura, & Parrill, 1977). The hysteria scale reflects somatic complaints. People scoring high for hysteria tend to maintain a façade of being well adjusted, which breaks down under stress, resulting in physical symptoms as an expression of distress. Exner et al.'s (1977) findings are unexpected, given that higher social class is typically associated with scoring higher rather than lower on hysteria.

Personality Disorders

Some research has examined personality characteristics among women who sell sex. Perhaps the most common observation is that women who sell sex are higher than comparison groups in impulsivity and sensation seeking (e.g., O'Sullivan, Zuckerman, & Kraft, 1996). A greater amount of research has examined links between selling sex and personality disorders. Personality disorders consist of enduring patterns of inner experiences and behaviors that deviate from the expectations in an individual's culture. They involve some combination of distorted thinking, problematic emotional responses, problems with impulse control, and interpersonal difficulties. They tend to manifest as inflexible responses to personal and social situations that are deeply ingrained and endure across time. In countries where selling sex is illegal or highly stigmatized, this activity may be more strongly linked to personality disorders, given that a feature of personality disorders includes deviating from sociocultural norms.

The most commonly studied personality disorder on this topic is antisocial personality disorder, likely because of the stereotype that selling sex is an antisocial behavior. Antisocial personality disorder involves a personal style that emphasizes ego-centrism, personal gain, power, and pleasure over conforming to laws or social norms. Individuals with antisocial personality disorder tend to lack empathy, including a lack of remorse when mistreating others, and their interactions with others may be based on exploitation rather than intimacy. Antisocial personality disorder may also involve psychopathic features, which can include a sense of boldness, attention seeking, or fearless dominance.

Research on links between antisocial personality disorder and selling sex has focused nearly exclusively on samples of women who abuse substances or have been involved in crimes. Research among substance abusing women has typically shown links between selling sex and antisocial personality disorder. Those with a diagnosis of antisocial personality disorder are more likely to have a lifetime history of ever having received money for sex (71 vs. 45% in Compton, Cottler, Shillington, & Price, 1995; 40 vs. 3% in Gill, Nolimal, & Crowley, 1992). Along similar lines, Edwards and Verona (2016) found among a sample of community dwelling women with a history of substance use and/or violence that antisocial characteristics were predictive of selling sex. Interestingly, when controlling for the intercorrelations between a number of features of antisocial personality disorder and psychopathy, callousness and lack of empathy were related to a lower likelihood of selling sex. They theorized that callousness and lack of empathy were likely associated with using more direct force to obtain money or goods, for example, through conning, stealing, and other ways of taking advantage of people, rather than relying on selling sex, which comparatively puts women in a more vulnerable position. An alternative explanation is that women higher in empathy may be more successful at selling sex, given the emotional labor involved.

Among a sample of female offenders, Edwards and Verona (2016) found that the impulsivity and irresponsibility characteristic of antisocial personality disorder were predictive of selling sex, even more so than drug dependence and cocaine use, which are common contributors to selling sex. They theorized that women high in impulsivity are less likely to consider the risks associated with selling sex and that those high in irresponsibility may turn to selling sex because they have challenges maintaining conventional work.

Although the research noted has found that women who sell sex are characterized by more antisocial personality traits than comparison groups, some research has shown this link can be attributed to differences in demographic factors. For example, O'Sullivan et al. (1996) found that a sample of women selling sex scored higher for aggression and hostility than a control group only when differences in age and education between the two groups were not taken into account. Similarly, the link between antisocial personality disorder and selling sex may be explained by substance abuse, which has independently been associated with sensation seeking and antisocial personality characteristics.

Beyond antisocial personality disorder, one study has linked the odd, eccentric cluster of personality disorders to selling sex among nonpsychotic incarcerated women (Warren et al., 2002). The common features of the odd, eccentric personality disorders are social awkwardness and social withdrawal. The researchers questioned whether the social isolation characteristic of this cluster of personality disorders may contribute to women being drawn to anonymous sexual activity or to selling sex as an alternative to more conventional relationships. Another possibility is that women who are eccentric or socially awkward turn to selling sex after finding it challenging to secure and maintain a conventional job requiring more social skills. When selling sex, eccentricity is often tolerated, and even celebrated.

Psychotic Disorders

Psychotic disorders are major mental illnesses that involve abnormal thinking or perceptions. Those with psychotic disorders may lose touch with reality through delusions or hallucinations. Not much work has focused on potential links between selling sex and psychotic disorders, and among the studies that have been conducted, the findings are somewhat mixed. In a study making use of a matched comparison group, women recruited from a hospital setting with a schizophrenia-spectrum disorder, including schizophrenia and schizoaffective disorder, were more likely than matched control participants without major mental illness to report that they had ever sold sex (23 vs. 2%, Miller & Finnerty, 1996). Along the same lines, among samples of female criminal offenders, those who had ever sold sex were more likely to have a diagnosis of schizophrenia than those who had never sold sex (Perdue et al., 2012). However, in another study, having a psychotic disorder was unrelated to whether or not a woman had traded sex for money, food, shelter, or drugs (DeHart et al., 2014).

Clearly, more research is needed to draw strong conclusions on this topic. The available research tentatively suggests there may be a link between psychotic disorders and selling sex. If so, one possibility is that women with psychotic disorders sell sex in response to various life challenges. This highlights the fact that some vulnerable populations are more likely to become involved in selling sex than those without similar vulnerabilities.

Discussion

Based on the research reviewed in this chapter, are links between selling sex and mental health concerns myth or fact? Those looking for a simple answer may be disappointed, as this question requires a nuanced response. The research literature shows that for many mental health concerns, women who sell sex demonstrate considerably higher prevalence compared to women in the general population, and in some cases also higher rates than in somewhat similar comparison groups. As acknowledged, prevalence of a particular disorder in the general population can be used as a general reference point, but the general population is typically not an appropriate reference group for women who sell sex. An ideal comparison group would closely match a sex-selling sample in demographic characteristics and all circumstances outside of selling sex. Although extremely valuable, this type of research is difficult to conduct and quite rare. When appropriate comparison groups are used, the differences in prevalence of mental health concerns between women who sell sex and women who do not sell sex are smaller in magnitude.

The increased prevalence of mental health concerns observed in the literature among women who sell sex does not establish whether selling sex is causally related to mental health concerns. Mental health concerns can be the result of many factors, such as poverty, discrimination, and violence, which may be related directly, indirectly, or not at all to selling sex for particular women. In addition, many mental health disorders are comorbid, meaning women who sell sex experience multiple mental health conditions simultaneously. For example, child sexual abuse and drug use both substantially increase the risk of suicidal behavior. These factors may, at least in part, contribute to the high prevalence of suicidal ideation and attempts that has been observed in certain samples of women selling sex. To attribute the high rate of suicidality solely to selling sex without acknowledging other factors would be inappropriate. Despite this, a simplistic approach is sometimes adopted in an attempt to persuade others that selling sex is harmful. Although perhaps well intentioned, inaccurate or incomplete arguments ultimately distract from stakeholders' efforts and abilities to aid women who sell sex and have mental health concerns. We believe prioritizing the welfare and mental health of women who sell sex must involve a pursuit of accurate information through high-quality research.

Despite the noted caveats, current research offers clear indications that many women who sell sex have experiences that can increase the likelihood of developing mental health problems, or can exacerbate pre-existing ones. For example, experiencing physical or sexual violence when selling sex can increase the likelihood of developing PTSD and other mental health concerns. There is also evidence that, in some cases, women who have mental health problems are more likely to start selling sex. In her research on job mobility in the Australian indoor sex industry, Gilmour

(2016) noted that for some women with pre-existing mental health problems, selling sex is an attractive option because it offers flexibility that cannot be found in more traditional jobs. Her interviews with women selling sex illustrate this idea, for example:

> When I've had issues with my mental health, there's no other job that you can have that you can step away from when you need to, and maybe pick up a shift once a week to keep yourself going, whilst you're dealing with whatever it is, whatever angst is going on. (Sallie, Sect. 3.10)

This has significant implications for providing support to vulnerable populations who become involved in commercial sex, a topic we address in Chap. 7.

Finally, the literature reviewed in this chapter clearly shows that the context where sex is sold matters. The prevalence of many mental health concerns appears to be considerably higher when sex is sold on the street or under other high-stress circumstances. Although differentiating indoor venues from outdoor venues is useful, the distinction is a crude one. Indoor venues differ widely from one another, and significant differences in mental health concerns have been observed across different indoor venues. A more in-depth examination of the diverse environments in which sex is sold will help to increase our understanding of the complex relationship between selling sex and mental health.

References

Abelson, A., Lyons, C., Decker, M., Ketende, S., Mfochive Njindam, I., Fouda, G., … Baral, S. D. (2019). Lifetime experiences of gender-based violence, depression and condom use among female sex workers in Cameroon. *International Journal of Social Psychiatry, 65*(6), 445–457. https://doi.org/10.1177/0020764019858646

Agaibi, C. E., & Wilson, J. P. (2005). Trauma, PTSD, and resilience: A review of the literature. *Trauma, Violence, & Abuse, 6,* 195–216. https://doi.org/10.1177/1524838005277438.

Akcali, N., Nazlican, E., Akbaba, M., & Kurt, B. (2017). Investigation of depression status of Adana brothel sex workers. *Sakarya Medical Journal, 7*(2), 85–91.

Alegría, M., Vera, M., Freeman, D. H., Robles, R., Santos, M. C., & Rivera, C. L. (1994). HIV infection, risk behaviors, and depressive symptoms among Puerto Rican sex workers. *American Journal of Public Health, 84,* 2000–2002. https://doi.org/10.2105/AJPH.84.12.2000.

Bellhouse, C., Crebbin, S., Fairley, C. K., & Bilardi, J. E. (2015). The impact of sex work on women's personal romantic relationships and the mental separation of their work and personal lives: A mixed-methods study. PLoS One, *10*(10). https://doi.org/10.1371/journal.pone.0141575.

Bilardi, J. E., Miller, A., Hocking, J. S., Keogh, L., Cummings, R., Chen, M. Y., et al. (2011). The job satisfaction of female sex workers working in licensed brothels in Victoria, Australia. *Journal of Sexual Medicine, 8,* 116–122. https://doi.org/10.1111/j.1743-6109.2010.01967.x.

Borges, G., & Loera, C. R. (2010). Alcohol and drug use in suicidal behaviour. *Current Opinion in Psychiatry, 23,* 195–204. https://doi.org/10.1097/YCO.0b013e3283386322.

Brunello, N., Davidson, J. T., Deahl, M., Kessler, R. C., Mendlewicz, J., Racagni, G., … Zohar, J. (2001). Posttraumatic stress disorder: Diagnosis and epidemiology, comorbidity and social consequences, biology and treatment. *Neuropsychobiology, 43,* 150–162. https://doi.org/10.1159/000054884.

Burnette, M. L., Lucas, E., Ilgen, M., Frayne, S. M., Mayo, J., & Weitlauf, J. C. (2008). Prevalence and health correlates of prostitution among patients entering treatment for substance use disorders. *Archives of General Psychiatry, 65,* 337–344. https://doi.org/10.1001/archpsyc.65.3.337.

Carlson, C. E., Witte, S. S., Pala, A. N., Tsai, L. C., Wainberg, M., & Aira, T. (2017). The Impact of Violence, Perceived Stigma, and Other Work-Related Stressors on Depressive Symptoms Among Women Engaged in Sex Work. *Global Social Welfare, 4*(2), 51–57. https://doi.org/10.1007/s40609-017-0085-5

Choi, H., Klein, C., Shin, M., & Lee, H. (2009). Posttraumatic stress disorder (PTSD) and disorders of extreme stress (DESNOS) symptoms following prostitution and childhood abuse. *Violence Against Women, 15,* 933–951. https://doi.org/10.1177/1077801209335493.

Chudakov, B., Ilan, K., Belmaker, R. H., & Cwikel, J. (2002). The motivation and mental health of sex workers. *Journal of Sex and Marital Therapy, 28,* 305–315. https://doi.org/10.1080/00926230290001439.

Clarke, R. J., Clarke, E. A., Roe-Sepowitz, D., & Fey, R. (2012). Age at entry into prostitution: Relationship to drug use, race, suicide, education level, childhood abuse, and family experiences. *Journal of Human Behavior in the Social Environment, 22,* 270–289. https://doi.org/10.1080/10911359.2012.655583.

Coetzee, J., Buckley, J., Otwombe, K., Milovanivic, M., Gray, G. E., & Jewkes, R. (2018). Depression and Post Traumatic Stress amongst female sex workers in Soweto, South Africa: A cross sectional, respondent driven sample. *PLoS One, 13*(7), e0196759. https://doi.org/10.1371/journal.pone.0196759.

Coleman, K. J., Stewart, C., Waitzfelder, B. E., Zeber, J. E., Morales, L. S., Ahmed, A. T., et al. (2016). Racial-ethnic differences in psychiatric diagnoses and treatment across 11 health care systems in the Mental Health Research Network. *Psychiatric Services, 67,* 749–757. https://doi.org/10.1176/appi.ps.201500217.

Compton, W. M., Cottler, L. B., Shillington, A. M., & Price, R. K. (1995). Is antisocial personality disorder associated with increased HIV risk behaviors in cocaine users? *Drug and Alcohol Dependence, 37,* 37–43. https://doi.org/10.1016/0376-8716(94)01056-Q.

Cwikel, J. J., Ilan, K. K., & Chudakov, B. B. (2003). Women brothel workers and occupational health risks. *Journal of Epidemiology and Community Health, 57,* 809–815. https://doi.org/10.1136/jech.57.10.809.

Daalder, A. L., Bogaerts, S., & Bijleveld, C. C. L. D. (2013). The severity of childhood abuse and neglect in relationship to post-traumatic stress disorder among female sex workers in the Netherlands. *Journal of Aggression, Maltreatment & Trauma, 22,* 935–949. https://doi.org/10.1080/10926771.2013.834017.

De Schampheleire, D. (1990). MMPI characteristics of professional prostitutes: A cross-cultural replication. *Journal of Personality Assessment, 54,* 343–350. https://doi.org/10.1207/s15327752jpa5401&2_31.

DeHart, D., Lynch, S., Belknap, J., Dass-Brailsford, P., & Green, B. (2014). Life history models of female offending: The roles of serious mental illness and trauma in women's pathways to jail. *Psychology of Women Quarterly, 38,* 138–151. https://doi.org/10.1177/0361684313494357.

Edwards, B. G., & Verona, E. (2016). Gendered contexts: Psychopathy and drug use in relation to sex work and exchange. *Journal of Abnormal Psychology, 125,* 514–527. https://doi.org/10.1037/abn0000159.

El-Bassel, N., Schilling, R. F., Irwin, K. L., Faruque, S., Gilbert, L., Von Bargen, J., … Edlin, B. R. (1997). Sex trading and psychological distress among women recruited from the streets of Harlem. *American Journal of Public Health, 87,* 66–70. https://doi.org/10.2105/AJPH.87.1.66.

El-Bassel, N., Simoni, J. M., Cooper, D. K., Gilbert, L., & Schilling, R. F. (2001). Sex trading and psychological distress among women on methadone. *Psychology of Addictive Behaviors, 15,* 177–184. https://doi.org/10.1037//0893-164X.15.3.177.

Eller, L., & Mahat, G. (2003). Psychological factors in Nepali former commercial sex workers with HIV. *Journal of Nursing Scholarship, 35,* 53–60. https://doi.org/10.1111/j.1547-5069.2003.00053.x.

Ellsberg, M., Jansen, H. M., Heise, L., Watts, C. H., & García-Moreno, C. (2008). Intimate partner violence and women's physical and mental health in the WHO multi-country study on women's health and domestic violence: An observational study. *The Lancet, 371*(9619), 1165–1172. https://doi.org/10.1016/S0140-6736(08)60522-X.

Exner, J. E. Jr., Wylie, J., Leura, A., & Parrill, T. (1977). Some psychological characteristics of prostitutes. *Journal of Personality Assessment, 41,* 474–485. https://doi.org/10.1207/s15327752jpa4105_3.

Farley, M., Cotton, A., Lynne, J., Zumbeck, S., Spiwak, F., Reyes, M. E., … Sezgin, U. (2003). Prostitution and trafficking in nine countries: An update on violence and posttraumatic stress disorder. *Journal of Trauma Practice, 2*(3/4), 33–74. https://doi.org/10.1300/j189v02n03_03.

Ghose, T., Chowdhury, A., Solomon, P., & Ali, S. (2015). Depression and anxiety among HIV positive sex workers in Kolkata, India: Testing and modifying the Hospital Anxiety Depression Scale. *International Social Work, 58*(2), 211–222. https://doi.org/10.1177/0020872813497381.

Gilchrist, G., Gruer, L., & Atkinson, J. (2005). Comparison of drug use and psychiatric morbidity between prostitute and non-prostitute female drug users in Glasgow, Scotland. *Addictive Behaviors, 30,* 1019–1023. https://doi.org/10.1016/j.addbeh.2004.09.003.

Gill, K., Nolimal, D., & Crowley, T. J. (1992). Antisocial personality disorder, HIV risk behavior and retention in methadone maintenance therapy. *Drug and Alcohol Dependence, 30,* 247–252. https://doi.org/10.1016/0376-8716(92)90059-L.

Gilmour, F. E. (2016). Work conditions and job mobility in the Australian indoor sex industry. *Sociological Research Online, 21*(4), 14. https://doi.org/10.5153/sro.4166.

Harvard Medical School. (2007a, July 19). *National Comorbidity Survey*. Table 2. 12-month prevalence of DSM-IV/WMH-CIDI disorders by sex and cohort. Retrieved from http://www.hcp.med.harvard.edu/ncs/ftpdir/NCS-R_12-month_Prevalence_Estimates.pdf.

Harvard Medical School. (2007b, July 19). *National Comorbidity Survey*. Table 1. Lifetime prevalence of DSM-IV/WMH-CIDI disorders by sex and cohort. Retrieved from http://www.hcp.med.harvard.edu/ncs/ftpdir/NCS-R_Lifetime_Prevalence_Estimates.pdf.

Hong, Y., Li, X., Fang, X., & Zhao, R. (2007). Correlates of suicidal ideation and attempt among female sex workers in China. *Health Care for Women International, 28,* 490–505. https://doi.org/10.1080/07399330701226529.

Hong, Y., Fang, X., Li, X., Liu, Y., Li, M., & Tai-Seale, T. (2010). Self-perceived stigma, depressive symptoms, and suicidal behaviors among female sex workers in China. *Journal of Transcultural Nursing, 21,* 29–34. https://doi.org/10.1177/1043659609349063.

Iaisuklang, M. G., & Ali, A. (2018). Psychiatric morbidity among female commercial sex workers. *Indian Journal of Psychiatry, 59,* 465–470. https://doi.org/10.4103/psychiatry.IndianJPsychiatry_147_16.

Jana, S., Ray, S., Roy, S., Piduttia, J., Ghose, T., & Jana, S. (2017). Depression and its relation with HIV risk and social well-being among the brothel-based female sex workers in Kolkata, India. *HSOA Journal of Community Medicine and Public Health Care, 4,* 25. https://doi.org/10.24966/CMPH-1978/100025.

Johnson, J. G., Cohen, P., Kasen, S., & Brook, J. S. (2006). Dissociative disorders among adults in the community, impaired functioning, and axis I and II comorbidity. *Journal of Psychiatric Research, 40,* 131–140. https://doi.org/10.1016/j.jpsychires.2005.03.003.

Jung, M. (2013). Associations of physical and sexual health with suicide attempts among female sex workers in South Korea. *Sexuality and Disability, 31,* 275–286. https://doi.org/10.1007/s11195-013-9305-9.

Jung, Y. E., Song, J. M., Chong, J., Seo, H., & Chae, J. (2008). Symptoms of posttraumatic stress disorder and mental health in women who escaped prostitution and helping activists in shelters. *Yonsei Medical Journal, 49,* 372–382. https://doi.org/10.3349/ymj.2008.49.3.372.

Kessler, R. C., Angermeyer, M., Anthony, J. C., De Graaf, R., Demyttenaere, K., Gasquet, I., … Uston, T. B. (2007). Lifetime prevalence and age-of-onset distributions of mental disorders in the World Health Organization's Mental Health Survey Initiative. *World Psychiatry, 6,* 168–176.

Koken, J. (2012). Independent female escort's strategies for coping with sex work related stigma. *Sexuality & Culture, 16,* 209–229. https://doi.org/10.1007/s12119-011-9120-3.

Kramer, L. A. (2003). Emotional experiences of performing prostitution. *Journal of Trauma Practice, 2,* 187–197. https://doi.org/10.1300/j189v02n03_10.

Lau, J. F., Tsui, H. Y., Ho, S. Y., Wong, E., & Yang, X. X. (2010). Prevalence of psychological problems and relationships with condom use and HIV prevention behaviors among Chinese female sex workers in Hong Kong. *AIDS Care, 22,* 659–668. https://doi.org/10.1080/09540120903431314.

MacLean, S. A., Lancaster, K. E., Lungu, T., Mmodzi, P., Hosseinipour, M. C., Pence, B. W., et al. (2018). Prevalence and correlates of probable depression and post-traumatic stress disorder among female sex workers in Lilongwe, Malawi. *International Journal of Mental Health and Addiction, 16,* 150–163. https://doi.org/10.1007/s11469-017-9829-9.

Marchand, K., Oviedo-Joekes, E., Guh, D., Marsh, D. C., Brissette, S., & Schechter, M. T. (2012). Sex work involvement among women with long-term opioid injection drug dependence who enter opioid agonist treatment. *Harm Reduction Journal, 9.* https://doi.org/10.1186/1477-7517-9-8.

Miller, L. J., & Finnerty, M. (1996). Sexuality, pregnancy, and childrearing among women with schizophrenia-spectrum disorders. *Psychiatric Services, 47,* 502–506. https://doi.org/10.1176/ps.47.5.502.

Ortblad, K. F., Kibuuka Musoke, D., Ngabirano, T., Nakitende, A., Harling, G., Haberer, J. E., … Bärnighausen, T. (2019). The effect of HIV self-testing delivery models on female sex workers' sexual behaviors: A randomized controlled trial in urban Uganda. *AIDS and Behavior, 23,* 1225–1235. https://doi.org/10.1007/s10461-019-02393-z.

O'Sullivan, D. M., Zuckerman, M., & Kraft, M. (1996). The personality of prostitutes. *Personality and Individual Differences, 21,* 445–448. https://doi.org/10.1016/0191-8869(96)00053-0.

Patterson, T. L., Semple, S. J., Abramovitz, D., Harvey-Vera, A., Pines, H. A., Verdugo, S., … Strathdee, S. A. (2019). Impact of time perspectives on texting intervention to reduce HIV/STI transmission among female sex workers in Tijuana and Ciudad Juarez, Mexico. *Journal of Behavioral Medicine, 42,* 111–127. https://doi.org/10.1007/s10865-018-9948-1.

Perdue, T. R., Williamson, C., Ventura, L. A., Hairston, T. R., Osborne, L. T., Laux, J. M., … Nathan, V. M. (2012). Offenders who are mothers with and without experience in prostitution: Differences in historical trauma, current stressors, and physical and mental health differences. *Women's Health Issues, 22*(2), e195–e200. https://doi.org/10.1016/j.whi.2011.08.010.

Potter, K., Martin, J., & Romans, S. (1999). Early developmental experiences of female sex workers: A comparative study. *Australian and New Zealand Journal of Psychiatry, 33,* 935–940. https://doi.org/10.1046/j.1440-1614.1999.00655.x.

Rael, C. T., & Davis, A. (2017). Elevated depression symptoms and key associated factors in female sex workers and women living with HIV/AIDS in the Dominican Republic. *International Journal of STD and AIDS, 28,* 433–440. https://doi.org/10.1177/0956462416651374.

Ranjbar, F., Sadeghi-bazargani, H., Pishgahi, A., Nobari, O., Farahbakhsh, M., Farhang, S., et al. (2018). Mental health status among female sex workers in tabriz, iran. *Archives of Women's Mental Health.* https://doi.org/10.1007/s00737-018-0907-1.

Regier, D. A. (1990). Comorbidity of Mental Disorders With Alcohol and Other Drug Abuse. *JAMA, 264*(19), 2511. https://doi.org/10.1001/jama.1990.03450190043026.

Risser, J. M. H., Timpson, S. C., McCurdy, S. A., Ross, M. W., & Williams, M. L. (2006). Psychological correlates of trading sex for money among African American crack cocaine smokers. *American Journal of Drug and Alcohol Abuse, 32,* 645–653. https://doi.org/10.1080/00952990600919062.

Roe-Sepowitz, D. E., Hickle, K. E., & Cimino, A. (2012). The impact of abuse history and trauma symptoms on successful completion of a prostitution-exiting program. *Journal of Human Behavior in the Social Environment, 22,* 65–77. https://doi.org/10.1080/10911359.2011.598830.

Romans, S. E., Potter, K., Martin, J., & Herbison, P. (2001). The mental and physical health of female sex workers: A comparative study. *Australian and New Zealand Journal of Psychiatry, 35,* 75–80. https://doi.org/10.1046/j.1440-1614.2001.00857.x.

Ross, C. A., Farley, M., & Schwartz, H. L. (2003). Dissociation among women in prostitution. *Journal of Trauma Practice,* 2(3/4), 199–212. https://doi.org/10.1300/j189v02n03_11.

Ross, C. A., Anderson, G., Heber, S., & Norton, G. R. (1990). Dissociation and abuse among multiple-personality patients, prostitutes, and exotic dancers. *Hospital & Community Psychiatry, 41,* 328–330. https://doi.org/10.1176/ps.41.3.32.

Rössler, W. W., Koch, U. U., Lauber, C. C., Hass, A. K., Altwegg, M. M., Ajdacic-Gross, V. V., et al. (2010). The mental health of female sex workers. *Acta Psychiatrica Scandinavica, 122,* 143–152. https://doi.org/10.1111/j.1600-0447.2009.01533.x.

Roxburgh, A., Degenhardt, L., & Copeland, J. (2006). Posttraumatic stress disorder among female street-based sex workers in the greater Sydney area, Australia. *BMC Psychiatry, 6*(24). https://doi.org/10.1186/1471-244x-6-24.

Sanders, T. (2001). Female street sex workers, sexual violence, and protection strategies. *Journal of Sexual Aggression, 7*(1), 5–18. https://doi.org/10.1080/13552600108413318.

Sanders, T. (2004). A continuum of risk? The management of health, physical and emotional risks by female sex workers. *Sociology of Health & Illness, 26,* 557–574. https://doi.org/10.1111/j.0141-9889.2004.00405.x.

Sanders, T., Connelly, L., & King, L. J. (2016). On Our Own Terms: The Working Conditions of Internet-Based Sex Workers in the UK. *Sociological Research Online, 21*(4), 133–146. https://doi.org/10.5153/sro.4152

Şar, V., Akyüz, G., & Doğan, O. (2007). Prevalence of dissociative disorders among women in the general population. *Psychiatry Research, 149,* 169–176. https://doi.org/10.1016/j.psychres.2006.01.005.

Seib, C., Dunne, M. P., Fischer, J., & Najman, J. M. (2012). Predicting the job satisfaction of female sex workers in Queensland, Australia. *International Journal of Sexual Health, 24,* 99–111. https://doi.org/10.1080/19317611.2011.632073.

Substance Abuse and Mental Health Services Administration. (2017, September 7). *Results from the 2016 National Survey on Drug Use and Health: Detailed tables*. Retrieved from https://www.samhsa.gov/data/sites/default/files/NSDUH-DetTabs-2016/NSDUH-DetTabs-2016.pdf.

Suresh, G., Furr, L., & Srikrishnan, A. (2009). An assessment of the mental health of street-based sex workers in Chennai, India. *Journal of Contemporary Criminal Justice, 25,* 186–201. https://doi.org/10.4135/9788132114109.n16.

Surratt, H. L., Kurtz, S. P., Weaver, J. C., & Inciardi, J. A. (2005). The connections of mental health problems, violent life experiences, and the social milieu of the "stroll" with the HIV risk behaviors of female street sex workers. *Journal of Psychology & Human Sexuality, 17,* 23–44. https://doi.org/10.1300/j056v17n01_03.

Teixeira, A., & Oliveira, A. (2017). Exploratory study on the prevalence of suicidal behavior, mental health, and social support in female street sex workers in Porto, Portugal. *Health Care for Women International, 38,* 159–166. https://doi.org/10.1080/07399332.2016.1192172.

Tomura, M. (2009). A prostitute's lived experiences of stigma. *Journal of Phenomenological Psychology, 40,* 51–84. https://doi.org/10.1163/156916209X427981.

Ulibarri, M. D., Semple, S. J., Rao, S., Strathdee, S. A., Fraga-Vallejo, M. A., Bucardo, J., & … Patterson, T. L. (2009). History of abuse and psychological distress symptoms among female sex workers in two Mexico–U.S. border cities. *Violence and Victims, 24,* 399–413. https://doi.org/10.1891/0886-6708.24.3.399.

Valera, R. J., Sawyer, R. G., & Schiraldi, G. R. (2000). Violence and post traumatic stress disorder in a sample of inner city street prostitutes. *American Journal of Health Studies, 16,* 149–155.

Volkow, N. D. (2004). The reality of comorbidity: Depression and drug abuse. *Biological Psychiatry, 56,* 714–717. https://doi.org/10.1016/j.biopsych.2004.07.007.

Warren, J. I., Burnette, M., South, S. C., Chauhan, P., Bale, R., & Friend, R. (2002). Personality disorders and violence among female prison inmates. *Journal of the American Academy of Psychiatry and The Law, 30,* 502–509.

Weissman, M. M., Bland, R. C., Canino, G. J., Greenwald, S., Hwu, H.-G., Joyce, P. R. …Yeh, E.-K. (1999). Prevalence of suicide ideation and suicide attempts in nine countries. *Psychological Medicine, 29,* 9–17. https://doi.org/10.1017/s0033291798007867.

Winstead, B. A., & Sanchez, J. (2016). The role of gender, race, and class in psychopathology. In J. E. Maddux & B. A. Winstead (Eds.), *Psychopathology: Foundations for a contemporary understanding* (4th ed., pp. 76–96). Routledge/Taylor & Francis Group.

Zhang, C., Li, X., Chen, Y., Hong, Y., Shan, Q., Liu, W., et al. (2014). Alcohol and other drug use, partner violence, and mental health problems among female sex workers in southwest China. *Health Care for Women International, 35*, 60–73. https://doi.org/10.1080/07399332.2012.757317.

Chapter 5
Alcohol and Drug Use and Abuse Among Women Selling Sex

In this chapter, we review alcohol and drug use among women who sell sex, a topic that has been studied extensively within the research literature. We begin by discussing some of the challenges of measuring alcohol and drug use in the context of selling sex and then review research on the prevalence of alcohol and substance use. Next, we review research relevant to questions such as: Do women tend to use alcohol and substances more before or after starting to sell sex? Does one impact the other more strongly? What are the reasons that women who sell sex use alcohol and drugs? We conclude by discussing some of the correlates and consequences of alcohol and drug use in the context of selling sex.

Measuring Drug and Alcohol Use

One challenge in summarizing the empirical knowledge regarding the role of alcohol and illicit substances when selling sex is the diversity of usage categories that have been examined. Differences in prevalence estimates of alcohol and substance use and differences in outcomes associated with alcohol and substance use among women who sell sex depend, in part, on how alcohol and substance consumption is measured in the literature. The International Classification of Diseases (ICD-10) differentiates between use, abuse, and dependence when it comes to alcohol and substances. In May 2013, the American Psychiatric Association issued the 5th edition of the Diagnostic and Statistical Manual of Mental Disorders (DSM-5), which contains two, single diagnoses for alcohol use disorder and substance use disorder, each with sub-classifications for severity. However, previous editions of the DSM differentiated distinct disorders of dependence and abuse.

Most studies that have examined the relationship between selling sex and alcohol or drugs have focused on alcohol or substance *use* rather than determining whether study participants met established criteria for diagnoses of dependence or abuse,

E. Krumrei Mancuso and B. E. Postlethwaite, *Women Who Sell Sex*,
https://doi.org/10.1007/978-3-030-47027-2_5

which is a more complex assessment. Substance use can be measured on the basis of any use, amount of use, frequency of use, type of substance used, or some other criteria. To illustrate, some studies have examined general drug use (e.g., "Have you ever used drugs?") whereas other studies have focused on the use of specific or multiple drugs (e.g., "Have you ever used cocaine?" "Have you used marijuana within the last year?") or administration route (e.g., "Have you ever injected drugs?"). A small number of studies have been conducted at the event-level. In these studies, women who sold sex were asked about alcohol or drug use during specific events or sexual encounters. These distinctions are important, given that the level and specificity of measurement can impact relationships with other variables, and ultimately the findings of the research.

Prevalence

A high volume of studies have reported the prevalence of alcohol and drug use and abuse among women who sell sex. We will provide a brief overview of patterns that have emerged in this research.

Factors Associated with Alcohol use Prevalence

The literature indicates that alcohol is commonly consumed by women who sell sex. Table 5.1 shows the prevalence of alcohol use among women who sell sex from a select number of studies, with statistics for women in the general United States population as a basic reference. The prevalence of overall alcohol use among women selling sex is comparable to women in the United States population as a whole. A unique feature to women who sell sex is that multiple studies have reported they consume alcohol in the course of their work, such as while looking for customers, entertaining customers, or before sex. We have provided details on this in Table 5.1.

Li, Li, and Stanton (2010) conducted a comprehensive review of alcohol use among women who sell sex. Their review suggests that the lifetime prevalence of ever drinking alcohol among women who sell sex is between 81 and 100%, with some studies indicating that women selling sex tend to regularly drink in excess of recommended amounts. For example, in a large study of women selling sex in China, 55% of women selling sex were identified as problem drinkers. Of those, 61% were classified as risk drinkers, 23% were classified as heavy drinkers, and 16% were classified as hazardous drinkers (Chen et al., 2012). Some comparison studies have found the prevalence of alcohol use, abuse, or dependency to be higher among women who sell sex than peer groups who do not sell sex. For example, women selling sex in South Africa were significantly more likely to have an alcohol dependency disorder

Table 5.1 Prevalence of alcohol use among women selling sex and women in the general United States population

Study	Country	Venue	Sample size	Work-related alcohol use[a] (%)	Overall alcohol use (%)	Time frame
de Graaf et al. (1995)	Netherlands	Outdoor: Street	29	17		
		Indoor: Window	27	19		
		Indoor: Home	12	42		
		Indoor: Brothel	27	56		
		Indoor: Club	32	81		
Wang et al. (2007)	China	Indoor	454	29		
Patterson et al. (2019)	Mexico (Tijuana)	Mixed	141	36		Past month
Yadav et al. (2005)	Kenya	Indoor: Home	224		35	Daily
		Indoor: Nightclub	30		53	Daily
		Indoor: Bar	212		60	Daily
Akcali et al. (2017)	Turkey	Indoor	108		47	Current
Markosyan et al. (2007)	Armenia	Not reported	98	~50		
Mahapatra et al. (2013)	India	Mixed		54		
Patterson et al. (2019)	Mexico (Cd. Juarez)	Mixed	129	59		Past month
Wirtz et al. (2015)	Russia	Mixed		69		
Plant et al. (1990)	Scotland		101	80	92	Past week
Persaud et al. (1999)	Guyana	Mixed	124	88		
Nasirian et al. (2017)	Iran	Not available	99		50	Current

(continued)

Table 5.1 (continued)

Study	Country	Venue	Sample size	Work-related alcohol use[a] (%)	Overall alcohol use (%)	Time frame
Abelson et al. (2019)	Cameroon	Mixed	2163		73	Past year
Surratt (2007)	US Virgin Islands	Indoor	101		73	Past month
					81	Lifetime
Sharma et al. (2016)	India	Multiple	417		77	Past month
Inciardi et al. (2005)	USA	Outdoor	407		78	Past month
					97	Lifetime
Iaisuklang & Ali (2018)	India	Mixed	100		79	Current
Van Nunen et al. (2014)	Belgium	Outdoor: Street	106		68	Past month
					95	Lifetime
	Belgium	Indoor: Window	122		56	Past month
					89	Lifetime
	Belgium	Indoor: Private	137		81	Past month
					99	Lifetime
	Belgium	Indoor: Escort	40		83	Past month
					93	Lifetime
	Belgium	Indoor: Bar & Club	120[b]		88	Past month
					97	Lifetime
Comparison population: U.S. adult females (2016)						
Substance Abuse and Mental Health Services Administration (2017)[c]	USA		27,181		50	Past month
					66	Past year
					83	Lifetime

[a] Work-related alcohol use includes drinking while looking for customers, entertaining customers, or before sex with customers

[b] Van Nunen et al. (2014) included one transgender worker in the Bar & Club sample

[c] Data from the National Survey on Drug Use and Health (NSDUH) from the Substance Abuse and Mental Health Services Administration (SAMHSA), Tables 2.33B, 2.34B, and 2.35B

both in the past year and in their lifetime than their counterparts who did not sell sex (Wechsberg et al., 2009).

Alcohol use has been found to vary between venues in which sex is sold. As might be expected, some studies have found that women working in establishments that serve alcohol, such as bars and clubs, report drinking more than those working in other locations such as on the street, at home, in brothels, and at window brothels (Chersich et al., 2007; de Graaf, Vanwesenbeeck, & van Zessen, 1995; Yadav et al., 2005). In a large study of women selling sex in China, researchers categorized the women as working in entertainment venues (e.g., night clubs), personal service venues (e.g., massage parlors), or on the street (Chen, Li, Shen, Zhou, & Tang, 2015). Compared to women working on the street, those working in entertainment and personal service venues were more likely to drink risky amounts. Studies have indicated that some establishments encourage or even require women to drink, sometimes to promote the sale of alcohol (van Nunen et al., 2014; Rodríguez, Fuentes, Ramos-Lira, Gutiérrez, & Ruiz, 2014). Moreover, some women have reported that customers pressure them into drinking (van Nunen et al., 2014), sometimes to the point of unconsciousness (Izugbara, 2005; Panchanadeswaran et al., 2008). Women working in personal service venues are more likely than those working in other locations to drink due to pressure from customers or managers (Chen et al., 2015). Following bars and clubs that serve alcohol, street workers are more likely to drink alcohol before selling sex than women who work in non–bar establishments, such as massage parlors and brothels (Chiao, Morisky, Rosenberg, Ksobiech, & Malow, 2006).

Limited research has examined links between immigration status and alcohol consumption among women who sell sex. Bautista et al. (2008) observed that being an immigrant in Uruguay was associated with more use of alcohol than not being an immigrant. They contributed this to the socioeconomic contexts in which the women worked, with immigrant women working in predominantly poorer locations than nonimmigrant women. On the other hand, Platt and colleagues (2011) found that among women selling sex in the UK, being an immigrant from Eastern Europe or the Former Soviet Union was associated with a lower likelihood of being a problem drinker (47%) compared to being from the UK (73%). This may relate to the fact that the women who immigrated to sell sex were more motivated to make money for education or savings than women from the UK.

Factors Associated with Drug Use Prevalence and Severity

Women selling sex use a variety of drugs, especially marijuana, crack, cocaine, methamphetamine, and heroin. It is difficult to determine from the research literature whether reported substance use necessarily indicates problem use in terms of meeting criteria for substance abuse or dependence. The reliability of self-reported drug use is also something to be considered; women participating in research may not always openly report drug use, especially if drugs are illegal in their country of residence.

Because of this, it is difficult to determine the true amount of drug use, abuse, or dependence.

Table 5.2 shows the prevalence of drug use among women who sell sex from a number of studies, with statistics for women in the general United States population as a basic reference. Studies that targeted drug users or recruited from substance abuse treatment facilities were excluded from this table, as these would artificially inflate drug use prevalence. Overall, the literature indicates that women who sell sex tend to use drugs at rates higher than both the general population and specific comparison samples. For example, a study recruiting women from a clinic for sexually transmitted diseases found that drug use was more commonly reported by women who sold sex (86%) than by those who did not (23%; Potterat, Rothenberg, Muth, Darrow, & Phillips-Plummer, 1998). In like manner, a comparison among female jail detainees[1] showed that drug use was significantly higher among women who sold sex than among those who did not (McClanahan, McClelland, Abram, & Teplin, 1999). In this study, women with moderate or severe cocaine or opiate use were much more likely than women who did not use these drugs to have sold sex (53 vs. 14%). A comparison study in South Africa found that in contrast to those who did not engage in commercial sex, women who sold sex reported more lifetime substance use for a number of drugs including cannabis, crack, cocaine, and heroin (Wechsberg et al., 2009).

Selling sex is linked not only to the prevalence of substance use, but also to the severity of substance use. Research has indicated that *heavier* drug use is predictive of selling sex or trading sex for drugs. For example, a large study of women from 22 locations throughout the United States who had used crack cocaine in the recent past indicated that both frequency and intensity of crack cocaine use was predictive of trading sex for money or drugs (Hoffman, Klein, Eber, & Crosby, 2000). Similarly, among a large sample of African American women who used crack cocaine, those who traded sex for money or drugs were more likely to have used crack heavily in the 30 days prior to the study, in comparison to those who had not traded sex (67 vs. 35%; Edwards, Halpern, & Wechsberg, 2006). Even when controlling for age, marital status, the number of friends who use drugs, childhood physical or sexual abuse, and PTSD, those who were heavy crack users were more likely to sell sex than those who used less crack.

The literature indicates that specific drug use among women who sell sex varies according to both geography—due to availability and legal status—as well as the venues in which sex is sold. Reported lifetime prevalence of any illicit drug use has ranged from 15% among women selling sex in a variety of settings in Iran (Sajadi et al., 2013) to 94% among women selling sex on the streets in Australia (Roxburgh, Degenhardt, & Copeland, 2006). Comparative studies have indicated that drugs are used more by women working on the street than in other venues (de Graaf et al., 1995; Odinokova, Rusakova, Urada, Silverman, & Raj, 2014). In a study from Belgium, women selling sex in window brothels reported lower usage of all types of drugs compared to women selling sex in bars and clubs, from home, or as an escort (van Nunen et al., 2014). These differences by venue may be due to the fact that indoor

[1] Mostly adults, but starting at age 17.

Table 5.2 Prevalence of illicit drug use among women selling sex and women in the general United States population

Study	Country	Venue	Sample size	Drug users (%)	Drug type	Timing
Overall drug use						
Abelson et al. (2019)	Cameroon	Mixed	2162	1	Any	Past year
Akcali et al. (2017)	Turkey	Indoor	108	3	Any	Current
Abelson et al. (2019)	Cameroon	Mixed	2162	10	Non-injection	Past year
Iaisuklang & Ali (2018)	India	Mixed	100	12	Cannabis	Current
Xu et al. (2013)	China	Mixed	1,642[a]	16	Any	Lifetime
Zhang et al. (2014)	China	Indoor	1022	18	Any	Lifetime
Medhi et al. (2012)	India		423	25	Any	Lifetime
Odinokova et al. (2014)	Russia (Orenburg)	Mixed	231	29	Any	Lifetime
				10	Any	Past 30 days
Platt et al. (2011)	UK (EE/FSU-Born)	Indoor	163	31	Any	Lifetime
Platt et al. (2011)	UK (EE/FSU-Born)	Indoor	105	58	Any	Lifetime
Teixeira & Oliveira (2017)	Portugal	Outdoor	52	33	Any	Current
Patterson et al. (2019)	Mexico (Tijuana)	Mixed	141	54	Non-injection heavy drugs	Past month
Patterson et al. (2019)	Mexico (Cd. Juarez)	Mixed	129	71	Non-injection heavy drugs	Past month
Kamel-Khodabandeh et al. (2018)	Iran	Outdoor	872	72	Any	Lifetime
Sajadi et al. (2013)	Iran	Mixed	871	74	Any	Lifetime
Odinokova et al. (2014)	Russia (St. Petersburg)	Mixed	665	86	Any	Lifetime
				74	Any	Past 30 Days
Van Nunen et al. (2014)	Belgium	Indoor/Window	122	18	Cannabis	Past month
				36		Lifetime
				10	Cocaine	Past month
				26		Lifetime
				1	Ecstasy	Past month
				16		Lifetime
				2	Amphet.	Past month
				16		Lifetime
				1	Crack	Past month

(continued)

Table 5.2 (continued)

Study	Country	Venue	Sample size	Drug users (%)	Drug type	Timing
				3		Lifetime
				0	Heroin[c]	Past month
				3		Lifetime
	Belgium	Indoor/Private	137	29	Cannabis	Past month
				68		Lifetime
				15	Cocaine	Past month
				46		Lifetime
				3	Ecstasy	Past month
				42		Lifetime
				5	Amphet.	Past month
				30		Lifetime
				1	Crack	Past month
				7		Lifetime
				1	Heroin[c]	Past month
				9		Lifetime
	Belgium	Indoor/Escort	40	13	Cannabis	Past month
				53		Lifetime
				8	Cocaine	Past month
				48		Lifetime
				10	Ecstasy	Past month
				48		Lifetime
				10	Amphet.	Past month
				38		Lifetime
				3	Crack	Past month
				5		Lifetime
				0	Heroin[c]	Past month
				13		Lifetime
	Belgium	Indoor/Bar & Club	120[b]	21	Cannabis	Past month
				60		Lifetime
				18	Cocaine	Past month

(continued)

Table 5.2 (continued)

Study	Country	Venue	Sample size	Drug users (%)	Drug type	Timing
				47		Lifetime
				0	Ecstasy	Past month
				38		Lifetime
				3	Amphet.	Past month
				25		Lifetime
				2	Crack	Past month
				3		Lifetime
				1	Heroin[c]	Past month
				9		Lifetime
	Belgium	Outdoor/Street	106	36	Cannabis	Past month
				72		Lifetime
				28	Cocaine	Past month
				63		Lifetime
				0	Ecstasy	Past month
				32		Lifetime
				4	Amphet.	Past month
				33		Lifetime
				11	Crack	Past month
				22		Lifetime
				34	Heroin[c]	Past month
				47		Lifetime
Injection drug use						
Odinokova et al. (2014)	Russia (Orenburg)	Mixed	231	2	Any	Past day
Sajadi et al. (2013)	Iran	Mixed	871	15	Any	Lifetime
Decker et al. (2012)	Russia	Mixed	147	18	Any	Lifetime
Strathdee et al. (2008)	Mexico	Mixed	924	18	Any	Lifetime
Markosyan et al. (2007)	Armenia	Street	98	19	Any	Lifetime
Hoffman et al. (2011)	Vietnam	Indoor	50	24	Opiates	Current

(continued)

Table 5.2 (continued)

Study	Country	Venue	Sample size	Drug users (%)	Drug type	Timing
Patterson et al. (2019)	Mexico (Tijuana)	Mixed	141	26	Any	Past month
Patterson et al. (2019)	Mexico (Cd. Juarez)	Mixed	129	46	Any	Past month
Nhurod et al. (2010)	Thailand	Indoor	236	27	Any	Lifetime
Nhurod et al. (2010	Thailand	Outdoor	83	40	Any	Lifetime
Alegría et al. (1994)	Puerto Rico	Mixed	127	47	Any	
Odinokova et al. (2014)	Russia (St. Petersburg)	Mixed	665	64	Any	Past day
Roxburgh et al. (2006)	Australia	Outdoor	72	94	Any	Lifetime
				83	Heroin	Past month
				42	Cocaine	Past month
Comparison population: U.S. adult females (2016), illicit drug use						
Substance Abuse and Mental Health Services Administration, (2017)[d]			27,181	9	Any	Past month
				15	Any	Past year
				47	Any	Lifetime

[a]Some of Xu et al.'s (2013) participants were as young as 16 years
[b]Van Nunen et al. (2014) included one transgender worker in the Bar & Club sample
[c]Heroin is frequently injected, but can also be smoked or snorted. The administration route was not specified
[d]Data from the National Survey on Drug Use and Health (NSDUH) from the Substance Abuse and Mental Health Services Administration (SAMHSA), Tables 1.29B, 1.30B, and 1.31B

establishments in some areas discourage drug use on the premises or may refuse to employ drug dependent women (Sanders & Campbell, 2007). However, a full range of policies exists. The managers in some clubs show zero tolerance toward illegal drug use, whereas other managers supply drugs and encourage or even force women to use drugs (van Nunen et al., 2014). Types of drugs used also differ by setting. In Belgium, women selling sex on the street are typically more likely to use crack or heroin, whereas women selling sex indoors are more likely to use ecstasy (van Nunen et al., 2014).

Immigrant status is a factor that has complex associations with the prevalence of substance abuse in interaction with setting. Bautista et al. (2008) observed that being an immigrant was associated with more drug use among women selling sex in Ecuador, whereas in Argentina, the opposite was true. Bautista et al. (2008) ascribed these differences to the socioeconomic contexts in which these women worked, with nonimmigrant women selling sex in Argentina being involved with more drug using customers than immigrant women selling sex there.

Platt et al. (2011) compared drug usage among women selling sex indoors in London on the basis of whether they were born in the United Kingdom or born in

Eastern Europe (EE) or the Former Soviet Union (FSU). Women born in the UK were more likely to have used drugs right before or while selling sex within the last four weeks than the EE/FSU-born women (28 vs. 11%). Platt and colleagues noted that compared to UK-born women, EE/FSU-born women in their sample were younger (Mean Age = 25 vs. 34) and their financial reasons for starting to sell sex were more likely to be studies or savings (31 vs. 13%) rather than drugs (0 vs. 10%).

Taken together, some samples of women who sell sex exhibit high rates of drug use. Unfortunately, women who sell sex and perceive that they have a substance use problem may face barriers in pursuing treatment (e.g., lack of education about programs, stigma) that may prevent them from receiving help (Wechsberg et al., 2009).

Timing: Which Tends to Come First, Substance Use or Selling Sex?

Many studies have examined samples of women who use drugs and sell sex. Table 5.3 provides a summary of a number of studies that report the timing regarding the order of onset of substance abuse versus selling sex. The studies in this table assessed substance abuse, addiction, or injection drug use. The majority of these studies report more frequent substance abuse/addiction prior to the first occurrence of selling sex than vice versa. An early study indicated that when comparing groups of women who

Table 5.3 Timing of initiation of selling sex and substance abuse among samples of drug-using women engaged in commercial sex

Study	% of sample who abused substances prior to beginning to sell sex	% of sample who sold sex before abusing substances	% of sample who concurrently started abusing drugs and selling sex
Morris et al. (2013)[a]	29	46	24
James (1976)	48	38	14
Roxburgh et al. (2006)[a]	53	26	Not specified
Silbert et al. (1982)[b]	55	30	15
McClanahan et al. (1999)[c]	67	22	10[d]
Potterat et al. (1998)	75 (injected drugs) 94 (noninjectable drugs)		

[a]Percentages for Morris et al. (2013) and Roxburgh et al. (2006) reflect injection drug use
[b]Silbert et al.'s (1982) sample included minors. The age range of the sample was 10–46 years, with an average of 22 years
[c]McClanahan et al. (1999) examined women who sold sex on a regular basis, defined as at least once per week and women who had a moderate to severe problem with cocaine or heroin
[d]Includes women who were uncertain about which behavior started first

sold sex first or used drugs first, a longer time span existed between starting to sell sex and the onset of addiction than between the onset of addiction and subsequently selling sex (James, 1976). Thus, it seemed to take longer for a woman who sold sex to move into addiction than for a woman addicted to drugs to start selling sex, although age differences between the groups may have played a factor in this pattern. James' (1976) ethnographic observations supported the idea that a woman addicted to substances would quickly turn to selling sex as a source of money, whereas forming a professional identity surrounding selling sex provided somewhat of a barrier against becoming addicted to drugs. Similarly, in a study of heavy drinking and drug using women, a path model indicated that cocaine dependence was predictive of trading sex for money, drugs, or other goods (Vaddiparti et al., 2006). Interestingly, other research has indicated that substance abuse does not impact entry into commercial sex. For example, research among female jail detainees (mostly adults, but starting at age 17) making use of an event-history analysis indicated that drug abuse did not affect when women started selling sex (McClanahan et al., 1999).

In considering findings regarding the ordering of selling sex and substance abuse, special consideration must be taken regarding the particular substances assessed in research. For example, a large study of crack smoking women selling sex in Miami, New York, and San Francisco, highlights that the median age of first having sex for money was 19 years and the median age of first crack use was 20 years (Jones et al., 1998). Thus, as a whole, the women in this study tended to have sold sex before they first smoked crack. However, it is important to understand that crack cocaine was not widely marketed in the neighborhoods where this study was conducted until around the median year when these women began selling sex, thus, some of the study participants first sold sex before crack cocaine was a viable option. Such considerations must be taken into account when trying to tease apart the question of time ordering.

Of note, as illustrated by Table 5.3, is that all samples included women who used substances before selling sex, women who sold sex before using substances, and women who initiated substance use and selling sex around the same time. Although we've noted studies emphasizing the route from substance abuse to selling sex, the literature has also highlighted that for some women, the stressors involved in selling sex and the availability of drugs in street-level contexts and certain indoor venues result in the initiation of substance use and abuse.

Another important consideration is that, even in circumstances where the relationship between initiating selling sex and initiating substances use is not causal in nature, they may become reinforcing of one another over time. Research has indicated that women who use illicit substances become *heavier* users if they start selling sex. Young, Boyd, and Hubbel (2000) reasoned that women who started selling sex to support drug use may *increase* their drug use as a means of coping with psychological distress caused by activities associated with selling sex. They found among urban, crack-addicted women that those who sold sex were addicted to a greater number of drugs than those who did not sell sex. These findings remained significant after controlling history of sexual trauma. Young et al. (2000) concluded that selling sex and drug use likely form a self-perpetuating cycle in which the involvement in one leads to an increase in the other. This theory has been supported by other research, such as a study from Australia, where almost three-quarters of the sample (71%) reported their drug use increased after starting to sell sex (Roxburgh et al., 2006). Over half of the sample (52%) reported they sold sex to pay for drugs and nearly the same amount of women (53%) reported they used drugs to facilitate their selling sex, mainly in order to numb themselves so that they would not have to think about what they were doing or experience emotions while selling sex. In this study, 18% of women described a reciprocal relationship between selling sex and drugs, i.e., they sold sex to obtain drugs and used drugs to facilitate selling sex.

Violence and Homicide in Relation to Substance Use Among Women Who Sell Sex

Violence in Relation to Selling Sex and Substance Use

In the general population, the experience of violence is associated with alcohol and substance use (e.g., Devries et al., 2014). The same is true for women who sell sex. Violence seems to relate to the links between selling sex and substance use in a number of ways. First, the experience of childhood violence seems to be predictive of both substance abuse and selling sex. Some research has suggested that women who have been sexually abused as children may turn to substance abuse as a form of coping, and subsequently rely on sex trading as a way to fund their substance abuse. For example, cocaine dependence has been found to function as a partial mediator explaining links between the experience of childhood sexual abuse and sex trading in adulthood, meaning that having experienced childhood sexual abuse is predictive of cocaine dependence, which in turn is predictive of sex trading (Vaddiparti et al., 2006). This illustrates how selling sex and substance abuse may relate to one another because they are both outgrowths of another variable, in this case, history of victimization or trauma (e.g., Silbert, Pines, & Lynch, 1982).

A fairly extensive body of research has also supported links between the experience of violence while selling sex and the use of alcohol and substances. For example, among women selling sex in southern China who had been forced to have sex against their will in the past six months, 41% indicated they had used alcohol before having sex with customers, which was a higher rate than among women who sold sex but had not been raped in the previous six months (Wang et al., 2007). A similar pattern was observed among women selling sex in Kenya, where binge drinkers were significantly more likely than non-binge drinkers to have been raped by a customer (Chersich et al., 2007). Along the same lines, studies conducted in New York and Mexico indicated that women who had experienced violence while selling sex were more likely to use crack or cocaine than those who had not experienced violence while selling sex (El-Bassel, Witte, Wada, Gilbert, & Wallace, 2001; Rodríguez, Fuentes, Ramos-Lira, Gutiérrez, & Ruiz, 2014). In New York, physical or sexual abuse from customers was also associated with greater injection drug use (El-Bassel et al., 2001). In Mexico, physical, sexual, or emotional abuse from customers, other sex workers, owners or employees of commercial sex venues, and police were all associated with more alcohol use (Rodríguez et al., 2014). Similarly, in Russia, having experienced sexual coercion from the police was associated with binge alcohol drinking among women selling sex (Odinokova, Rusakova, Urada, Silverman, & Raj, 2014).

There are multiple explanations for these findings. A salient possibility is that the experience of violence while selling sex contributes to women relying on alcohol and drugs more often when selling sex, as a coping mechanism to reduce painful memories of abuse. In addition, women who drink or use substances may also be more vulnerable to sexual abuse while selling sex. For example, in a sample of women selling sex in Belgium, 21% reported that taking drugs made them less selective in the customers they accepted (Van Nunen, et al., 2014). This may make these women more vulnerable to violent customers. This is mirrored by experimental research in the general population, which has indicated that women who have consumed alcohol anticipate less risk related to sexual vulnerability and indicate a greater likelihood of engaging in sexually risky behaviors (Testa, Livingston, & Collins, 2000).

Further, research with college students has indicated that both victims and perpetrators have reported that alcohol and substances are used as methods to force sexual intercourse (for a review, see George & Stoner, 2000). Perpetrators of violence have been known to use alcohol or substances as a tool, encouraging or forcing the use among women selling sex (e.g., Wang et al., 2007). This can make women vulnerable not only to violence and abuse, but to other crimes such as theft, as illustrated by a woman selling sex in Nigeria (quoted in Izugbara, 2005, p. 149):

> I remember a day a man picked me up. He offered a good price… He took me to a bar and made me drink very heavily. He then took me to a hotel and had sex with me several times. I don't even know if he used condom because I'd passed out. I recovered much later in the day and he was gone and so were my trinkets, purse, shoes, and watch. If he intended to kill me, he would have. He didn't even pay me. If I hadn't taken all those drinks, maybe it wouldn't have happened. (Soma, age 31)

Homicide in Relation to Selling Sex and Substance Use

We note one additional correlate of concern in the relationship between selling sex and substance use, which is homicide. Brewer et al. (2006) noted an increase in homicides among women who sell sex and their customers beginning in the late 1980 and early 1990s which can potentially be attributed to a rise in the use of crack cocaine. Crack cocaine use can result in increased vulnerability and increased aggression, both of which can contribute to the likelihood of homicide among women who sell sex. For example, data from sex work-related homicides in 1988 in 33 urban US counties showed 82% (14/17) of victims were under the influence of cocaine at the time of the homicide (see Table 7 in Brewer et al., 2006). Similarly, 74% of victims of sex-work related homicides (51/69) between 1988 and mid-2000 were under the influence of cocaine (see Table 7 in Brewer et al., 2006).

Salfati, James, and Ferguson (2008) compared homicides of women who sold sex in the UK between 1990 and 2001 to other sexual and nonsexual homicides of women. They found that 94% (31/33) of homicides among women who sold sex had involved some form of substance abuse (alcohol, drugs, or solvents). However, the direct role, if any, that substance use played in their deaths was not reported. In a more recent study of homicide and selling sex in the UK (Cunningham, Sanders, Platt, Grenfell, & Macioti, 2018), the authors argued that a distinction should be made between homicides that occur while the victim is selling sex versus homicides that occur in other contexts. They refer to the former as "occupational homicide" and argue that classifying deaths in this manner will allow a better understanding of the circumstances surrounding homicides as well as more focused policy responses. These authors were unable to examine the role of drug use in the homicides in their database due to inconsistent inclusion of drug use data.

Why do Women Who Sell Sex Use Alcohol and Drugs?

In the previous sections, we reviewed a number of ways that women who sell sex can be involved with alcohol and substances, including by force or influence from customers or managers. We have also noted that alcohol and substances can be employed as coping mechanisms. In this section, we explore in more detail the potential motivating factors for the use of alcohol and substances among women who sell sex.

Coping

As noted, a theme in the research is that some women who sell sex use drugs or alcohol as a mechanism to cope with stressors associated with selling sex. Young, Boyd, and Hubbel (2000) found among crack-using women, that those who sold sex were more likely to report using drugs as a coping mechanism than those who did not sell sex. These findings remained even after controlling for history of sexual trauma.

Women have described using drugs or alcohol to reduce distress about selling sex, numb or suppress negative thoughts, memories, or emotions while selling sex, detach from themselves while selling sex, decrease feelings of guilt, gain a sense of confidence or control, and cope with fears associated with commercial sex, including fears of sexual or physical violence during encounters with customers and social fears and anxiety associated with stigmas (e.g., Chen, Li, Shen, Zhou, & Tang, 2015; Kramer, 2003; Morris et al., 2013; Roxburgh et al., 2006; Young et al., 2000).

To Facilitate Selling Sex

Alcohol and substances can be used to support selling sex in ways other than coping. For example, in a sample of women selling sex in Belgium, 56% indicated that being under the influence of drugs made selling sex easier for them, with women reporting that drugs made them more confident in negotiating with customers (37% of sample) and made it easier for them to reject customers (30% of sample; van Nunen, Leuridan, Van Hal, Van Damme, & Decorte, 2014). A study from China indicated that some women who sell sex use alcohol to become less inhibited or to enhance sex, which were both associated with problem drinking (Chen et al., 2015).

Peers

As is seen in the general population, some women who sell sex begin using drugs due to peer pressure (Morris et al., 2013). In a large study of women selling sex in China, perceived peer alcohol use was a strong predictor of problem drinking (Chen et al., 2015). For some women who sell sex, using substances is something to be shared with others that facilitates social connection (Murphy, 2010). This is likely enhanced by availability. Among some samples, women who have ever sold sex are more likely to live in an area with high drug activity than women who have never sold sex (Perdue et al., 2012).

Personality

As is seen in the general population, personality factors are predictive of drug use among women who sell sex. For example, higher levels of impulsivity and sensation seeking have been associated with cocaine and polydrug use among women who sell sex (O'Sullivan, Zuckerman, & Kraft, 1996).

Discussion

A large volume of research has examined alcohol and drug use and abuse among women who sell sex. In some studies, alcohol or substance use is the focal research question, in other research it constitutes one of many variables examined. Research that has assessed whether study participants have met established criteria for diagnoses of dependence or abuse is rare. More commonly, alcohol and substance use is assessed. This limits our ability to understand the extent and seriousness of the problem as well as the risks to the women involved. We observed great variance in how use was measured across studies. Different measurement methods make direct comparison between studies challenging.

Our review suggests that, in general, women who sell sex use alcohol and drugs at higher proportions than women in the general population, or at least the population of United States adult females that was used for comparison. As was the case for mental health concerns presented in Chap. 4, the literature reviewed in this chapter clearly shows that the context where sex is sold matters. There is great variation in alcohol and drug use prevalence between studies of women selling sex, and factors such as work venue and geography help to explain some of this variance. Not surprisingly, alcohol use is higher in contexts where sex is sold in bars and nightclubs, businesses where alcohol is widely available and a prominent feature. On the other hand, drug use is higher among women selling sex on the street.

A common stereotype is that all women who sell sex use alcohol and drugs, and this contributes to negative stigma encountered by women selling sex. The prevalence data clearly refutes this notion—some women who sell sex use neither alcohol nor drugs. Further, those who use these substances do so at varying levels ranging from occasional recreational use to regular use, to use before and during sex with customers. The data is mixed with regard to whether or not selling sex leads to substance use, whether substance use leads to selling sex, or whether women begin selling sex and using drugs around the same time. Likely, each of these scenarios occur to some extent, with the most research evidence supporting a path from substance abuse to selling sex. Further, it appears that substance use and selling sex can be mutually reinforcing of one another over time.

Alcohol and drug use, and abuse, can adversely impact both mental and physical health. Likewise, women selling sex who use alcohol and drugs are at greater risk for becoming victims of sexual assault, violence, and in extreme circumstances, homicide. Given this, properly assessing and treating alcohol and substance use disorders among women selling sex should be a priority for helping professionals and policy makers. We discuss this further in Chap. 6, which addresses transitioning out of selling sex, and in Chap. 7, which contains information for mental health professionals working with women who sell sex or who have sold sex in the past.

References

Abelson, A., Lyons, C., Decker, M., Ketende, S., Mfochive Njindam, I., Fouda, G., et al. (2019). Lifetime experiences of gender-based violence, depression and condom use among female sex workers in Cameroon. *International Journal of Social Psychiatry, 65,* 445–457. https://doi.org/10.1177/0020764019858646.

Akcali, N., Nazlican, E., Akbaba, M., & Kurt, B. (2017). Investigation of depression status of Adana brothel sex workers. *Sakarya Medical Journal, 7*(2), 85–91.

Alegría, M., Vera, M., Freeman, D. H., Robles, R., Santos, M. C., & Rivera, C. L. (1994). HIV infection, risk behaviors, and depressive symptoms among Puerto Rican sex workers. *American Journal of Public Health, 84,* 2000–2002. https://doi.org/10.2105/AJPH.84.12.2000.

Bautista, C. T., Mosquera, C., Serra, M., Gianella, A., Avila, M. M., Laguna-Torres, V., … Sanchez, J. L. (2008). Immigration status and HIV-risk related behaviors among female sex workers in South America. *AIDS and Behavior, 12,* 195–201. https://doi.org/10.1007/s10461-007-9270-3.

Brewer, D. D., Dudek, J. A., Potterat, J. J., Muth, S. Q., Roberts, J. M., Jr., & Woodhouse, D. E. (2006). Extent, trends, and perpetrators of prostitution-related homicide in the United States. *Journal of Forensic Sciences, 51,* 1101–1108. https://doi.org/10.1111/j.1556-4029.2006.00206.x.

Chen, Y., Li, X., Shen, Z., Zhou, Y., & Tang, Z. (2015). Drinking reasons and alcohol problems by work venue among female sex workers in Guangxi, China. *Substance Use and Misuse, 50,* 642–652. https://doi.org/10.3109/10826084.2014.997827.

Chen, Y., Li, X., Zhou, Y., Zhang, C., Wen, X., & Guo, W. (2012). Alcohol consumption in relation to work environment and key sociodemographic characteristics among female sex workers in China. *Substance Use and Misuse, 47,* 1086–1099. https://doi.org/10.3109/10826084.2012.678540.

Chersich, M. F., Luchters, S. F., Malonza, I. M., Mwarogo, P., King'ola, N., & Temmerman, M. (2007). Heavy episodic drinking among Kenyan female sex workers is associated with unsafe sex, sexual violence and sexually transmitted infections. *International Journal of STD and AIDS, 18,* 764–769. https://doi.org/10.1258/095646207782212342.

Chiao, C., Morisky, D. E., Rosenberg, R., Ksobiech, K., & Malow, R. (2006). The relationship between HIV/sexually transmitted infection risk and alcohol use during commercial sex episodes: Results from the study of female commercial sex workers in the Philippines. *Substance Use and Misuse, 41,* 1509–1533. https://doi.org/10.1080/10826080600846284.

Cunningham, S., Sanders, T., Platt, L., Grenfell, P., & Macioti, P. G. (2018). Sex work and occupational homicide: Analysis of a U.K. murder database. *Homicide Studies, 22,* 321–338. https://doi.org/10.1177/1088767918754306.

de Graaf, R. D., Vanwesenbeeck, I., Zessen, G. V., Straver, C. J., & Visser, J. H. (1995). Alcohol and drug use in heterosexual and homosexual prostitution, and its relation to protection behaviour. *AIDS Care, 7,* 35–48. https://doi.org/10.1080/09540129550126948.

Decker, M. R., Wirtz, A. L., Baral, S. D., Peryshkina, A., Mogilnyi, V., Weber, R. A., … Beyrer, C. (2012). Injection drug use, sexual risk, violence, and STI/HIV among Moscow FSWs. *Sexually Transmitted Infections, 88,* 278–283. https://doi.org/10.1136/sextrans-2011-05017.

Devries, K. M., Child, J. C., Bacchus, L. J., Mak, J., Falder, G., Graham, K., … Heise, L. (2014). Intimate partner violence victimization and alcohol consumption in women: A systematic review and meta-analysis. *Addiction, 109,* 379–391. https://doi.org/10.1111/add.12393.

Edwards, J. M., Halpern, C. T., & Wechsberg, W. M. (2006). Correlates of exchanging sex for drugs or money among women who use crack cocaine. *AIDS Education and Prevention, 18,* 420–429. https://doi.org/10.1521/aeap.2006.18.5.420.

El-Bassel, N., Witte, S. S., Wada, T., Gilbert, L., & Wallace, J. (2001). Correlates of partner violence among female street-based sex workers: Substance abuse, history of childhood abuse, and HIV risks. *AIDS Patient Care and STDs, 15,* 41–51. https://doi.org/10.1089/108729101460092.

George, W. H., & Stoner, S. A. (2000). Understanding acute alcohol effects on sexual behavior. *Annual Review of Sex Research, 11,* 92–124.

Hoffman, J. A., Klein, H., Eber, M., & Crosby, H. (2000). Frequency and intensity of crack use as predictors of women's involvement in HIV-related sexual risk behaviors. *Drug and Alcohol Dependence, 58,* 227–236. https://doi.org/10.1016/s0376-8716(99)00095-2.

Hoffman, L., Nguyen, H. T. T., Kershaw, T. S., & Niccolai, L. M. (2011). Dangerous subtlety: Relationship-related determinants of consistency of condom use among female sex workers and their regular, non-commercial partners in Hai Phong, Viet Nam. *AIDS and Behavior, 15,* 1372–1380. https://doi.org/10.1007/s10461-010-9819-4.

Iaisuklang, M. G., & Ali, A. (2018). Psychiatric morbidity among female commercial sex workers. *Indian Journal of Psychiatry, 59,* 465–470. https://doi.org/10.4103/psychiatry.IndianJPsychiatry_147_16.

Inciardi, J. A., Surratt, H. L., Kurtz, S. P., & Weaver, J. C. (2005). The effect of serostatus on HIV risk behaviour change among women sex workers in Miami. *Florida. AIDS Care, 17*(sup1), 88–101. https://doi.org/10.1080/09540120500121011.

Izugbara, C. O. (2005). 'Ashawo suppose shine her eyes': Female sex workers and sex work risks in Nigeria. *Health, Risk & Society, 7,* 141–159. https://doi.org/10.1080/13698570500108685.

James, J. (1976). Prostitution and addiction: An interdisciplinary approach. *Addictive Diseases: An International Journal, 2,* 601–618.

Jones, D. L., Irwin, K. L., Inciardi, J., Bowser, B., Schilling, R., Word, C., ... Edlin, B. R. (1998). The high-risk sexual practices of crack-smoking sex workers recruited from the streets of three American cities. *Sexually Transmitted Diseases, 25,* 187–193. https://doi.org/10.1097/00007435-199804000-00002.

Kamel-Khodabandeh, A., Mirzaee, M., Jahani, Y., & Sharifi, H. (2018). Sex under influence of drugs: A nationwide survey among Iranian female sex workers. *Addiction & Health, 10*(4), 205–215. https://doi.org/10.22122/ahj.v10i4.566.

Kramer, L. A. (2003). Emotional experiences of performing prostitution. *Journal of Trauma Practice, 2,* 187–197. https://doi.org/10.1300/j189v02n03_10.

Li, Q., Li, X., & Stanton, B. (2010). Alcohol use among female sex workers and male clients: An integrative review of global literature. *Alcohol and Alcoholism, 45,* 188–199. https://doi.org/10.1093/alcalc/agp095.

Mahapatra, B., Lowndes, C. M., Mohanty, S. K., Gurav, K., Banadakoppa, M. R., Moses, S., ... Washington, R. (2013). Factors associated with risky sexual practices among female sex workers in Karnataka, India. *PLOS One, 8*(4), e62167. https://doi.org/10.1371/journal.pone.0062167.

Markosyan, K. M., Babikian, T., DiClemente, R. J., Hirsch, J. S., Grigoryan, S., & del Rio, C. (2007). Correlates of HIV risk and preventive behaviors in Armenian female sex workers. *AIDS and Behavior, 11,* 325–334. https://doi.org/10.1007/s10461-006-9147-x.

McClanahan, S. F., McClelland, G. M., Abram, K. M., & Teplin, L. A. (1999). Pathways into prostitution among female jail detainees and their implications for mental health service. *Psychiatric Services, 50,* 1606–1613. https://doi.org/10.1176/ps.50.12.1606.

Medhi, G. K., Mahanta, J., Kermode, M., Paranjape, R. S., Adhikary, R., Phukan, S. K., & Ngully, P. (2012). Factors associated with history of drug use among female sex workers (FSW) in a high HIV prevalence state of India. *BMC Public Health, 12*(1). https://doi.org/10.1186/1471-2458-12-273.

Morris, M. D., Lemus, H., Wagner, K. D., Martinez, G., Lozada, R., Gómez, R., et al. (2013). Factors associated with pathways toward concurrent sex work and injection drug use among female sex workers who inject drugs in northern Mexico. *Addiction, 108,* 161–170. https://doi.org/10.1111/j.1360-0443.2012.04016.x.

Murphy, L. (2010). Understanding the social and economic contexts surrounding women engaged in street-level prostitution. *Issues in Mental Health Nursing, 31,* 775–784. https://doi.org/10.3109/01612840.2010.524345.

Nasirian, M., Kianersi, S., Hoseini, S. G., Kassaian, N., Yaran, M., Shoaei, P., ... Jalilian, M. R. (2017). Prevalence of sexually transmitted infections and their risk factors among female sex workers in Isfahan, Iran: A cross-sectional Study. *Journal of the International Association of Providers of AIDS Care, 16,* 608–614. https://doi.org/10.1177/2325957417732836.

Nhurod, P., Bollen, L. J. M., Smutraprapoot, P., Suksripanich, O., Siangphoe, U., Lolekha, R., ... Fox, K. K. (2010). Access to HIV testing for sex workers in Bangkok, Thailand: A high prevalence of HIV among street-based sex workers. *Southeast Asian Journal of Tropical Medicine and Public Health, 41,* 153–162.

Odinokova, V., Rusakova, M., Urada, L. A., Silverman, J. G., & Raj, A. (2014). Police sexual coercion and its association with risky sex work and substance use behaviors among female sex workers in St. Petersburg and Orenburg, Russia. *International Journal of Drug Policy, 25,* 96–104. https://doi.org/10.1016/j.drugpo.2013.06.008.

O'Sullivan, D. M., Zuckerman, M., & Kraft, M. (1996). The personality of prostitutes. *Personality and Individual Differences, 21,* 445–448. https://doi.org/10.1016/0191-8869(96)00053-0.

Panchanadeswaran, S., Johnson, S. C., Sivaram, S., Srikrishnan, A. K., Latkin, C., Bentley, M. E., ... Celentano, D. (2008). Intimate partner violence is as important as client violence in increasing street-based female sex workers' vulnerability to HIV in India. *International Journal of Drug Policy, 19,* 106–112. https://doi.org/10.1016/j.drugpo.2007.11.013.

Patterson, T. L., Semple, S. J., Abramovitz, D., Harvey-Vera, A., Pines, H. A., Verdugo, S., … Strathdee, S. A. (2019). Impact of time perspectives on texting intervention to reduce HIV/STI transmission among female sex workers in Tijuana and Ciudad Juarez, Mexico. *Journal of Behavioral Medicine, 42,* 111–127. https://doi.org/10.1007/s10865-018-9948-1.

Perdue, T. R., Williamson, C., Ventura, L. A., Hairston, T. R., Osborne, L. T., Laux, J. M., … Nathan, V. M. (2012). Offenders who are mothers with and without experience in prostitution: Differences in historical trauma, current stressors, and physical and mental health differences. *Women's Health Issues, 22*(2), e195–e200. https://doi.org/10.1016/j.whi.2011.08.010.

Persaud, N. E., Klaskala, W., Tewari, T., Schultz, J., & Baum, M. (1999). Drug use and syphilis: Co-factors for HIV transmission among commercial sex workers in Guyana. *West Indian Med Journal, 48,* 52–56.

Plant, M. L., Plant, M. A., & Thomas, R. M. (1990). Alcohol, AIDS risks and commercial sex: Some preliminary results from a Scottish study. *Drug and Alcohol Dependence, 25,* 51–55. https://doi.org/10.1016/0376-8716(90)90141-z.

Platt, L., Grenfell, P., Bonell, C., Creighton, S., Wellings, K., Parry, J., et al. (2011). Risk of sexually transmitted infections and violence among indoor-working female sex workers in London: The effect of migration from Eastern Europe. *Sexually Transmitted Infections, 87,* 377–384. https://doi.org/10.1136/sti.2011.049544.

Potterat, J. J., Rothenberg, R. B., Muth, S. Q., Darrow, W. W., & Phillips-Plummer, L. (1998). Pathways to prostitution: The chronology of sexual and drug abuse milestones. *Journal of Sex Research, 35,* 333–340. https://doi.org/10.1080/00224499809551951.

Rodriguez, E. M., Fuentes, P., Ramos-Lira, L., Gutierrez, R., & Ruiz, E. (2014). Violencia en el entorno laboral del trabajo sexual y consumo de sustancias en mujeres mexicanas [Violence in the work environment of sex work and substance use in a group of Mexican women]. *Salud Mental, 37,* 355–360. https://doi.org/10.17711/sm.0185-3325.2014.041.

Roxburgh, A., Degenhardt, L., & Copeland, J. (2006). Posttraumatic stress disorder among female street-based sex workers in the greater Sydney area, Australia. *BMC Psychiatry*, *6*(24). https://doi.org/10.1186/1471-244X-6-24.

Sajadi, L., Mirzazadeh, A., Navadeh, S., Osooli, M., Khajehkazemi, R., Gouya, M. M., … Haghdoost, A. (2013). HIV prevalence and related risk behaviours among female sex workers in Iran: Results of the national biobehavioral survey, 2010. *Sexually Transmitted Infections, 89,* iii37–iii40. https://doi.org/10.1136/sextrans-2013-051028.

Salfati, C. G., James, A. R., & Ferguson, L. (2008). Prostitute homicides: A descriptive study. *Journal of Interpersonal Violence, 23,* 505–543. https://doi.org/10.1177/0886260507312946.

Sanders, T., & Campbell, R. (2007). Designing out vulnerability, building in respect: Violence, safety, and sex work policy. *British Journal of Sociology, 58,* 1–19. https://doi.org/10.1111/j.1468-4446.2007.00136.x.

Sharma, S. K., Singh, S. K., & Talukdar, B. (2016). Understanding the factors associated with alcohol use among female sex workers in a high HIV prevalence northeast state of India. *Journal of Infectious Diseases and Treatment, 1*(12). https://doi.org/10.21767/2472-1093.100017.

Silbert, M. H., Pines, A. M., & Lynch, T. (1982). Substance abuse and prostitution. *Journal of Psychoactive Drugs, 14,* 193–197. https://doi.org/10.1080/02791072.1982.10471928.

Strathdee, S. A., Philbin, M. M., Semple, S. J., Pu, M., Orozovich, P., Martinez, G., … & Patterson, T. L. (2008). Correlates of injection drug use among female sex workers in two Mexico–U.S. border cities. *Drug and Alcohol Dependence, 92,* 132–140. https://doi.org/10.1016/j.drugalcdep.2007.07.001.

Substance Abuse and Mental Health Services Administration. (2017, September 7). *Results from the 2016 National Survey on drug use and health: Detailed tables*. Retrieved from https://www.samhsa.gov/data/sites/default/files/NSDUH-DetTabs-2016/NSDUH-DetTabs-2016.pdf.

Surratt, H. (2007). Sex work in the Caribbean Basin: Patterns of substance use and HIV risk among migrant sex workers in the US Virgin Islands. *AIDS Care, 19,* 1274–1282. https://doi.org/10.1080/09540120701426490.

Teixeira, A., & Oliveira, A. (2017). Exploratory study on the prevalence of suicidal behavior, mental health, and social support in female street sex workers in Porto, Portugal. *Health Care for Women International, 38,* 159–166. https://doi.org/10.1080/07399332.2016.1192172.

Testa, M., Livingston, J. A., & Collins, R. L. (2000). The role of women's alcohol consumption in evaluation of vulnerability to sexual aggression. *Experimental and Clinical Psychopharmacology, 8,* 185–191. https://doi.org/10.1037/1064-1297.8.2.185.

Vaddiparti, K., Bogetto, J., Callahan, C., Abdallah, A. B., Spitznagel, E. L., & Cottler, L. B. (2006). The effects of childhood trauma on sex trading in substance using women. *Archives of Sexual Behavior, 35,* 451–459. https://doi.org/10.1007/s10508-006-9044-4.

van Nunen, K., Leuridan, E., Van Hal, G., Van Damme, P., & Decorte, T. (2014). Legal and illegal drug use among female sex workers in bar and club prostitution in Belgium: A qualitative and quantitative study. *Drugs: Education Prevention, and Policy, 21,* 56–64. https://doi.org/10.3109/09687637.2013.806432.

Wang, B., Li, X., Stanton, B., Fang, X., Yang, H., Zhao, R., et al. (2007). Sexual coercion, HIV-related risk, and mental health among female sex workers in China. *Health Care for Women International, 28,* 745–762. https://doi.org/10.1080/07399330701465226.

Wechsberg, W. M., Wu, L., Zule, W. A., Parry, C. D., Browne, F. A., Luseno, W. K., ... Gentry, A. (2009). Substance abuse, treatment needs and access among female sex workers and non-sex workers in Pretoria, South Africa. *Substance Abuse Treatment, Prevention & Policy, 4,* 11. https://doi.org/10.1186/1747-597X-4-11.

Wirtz, A. L., Peryshkina, A., Mogilniy, V., Beyrer, C., & Decker, M. R. (2015). Current and recent drug use intensifies sexual and structural HIV risk outcomes among female sex workers in the Russian Federation. *International Journal of Drug Policy, 26,* 755–763. https://doi.org/10.1016/j.drugpo.2015.04.017.

Xu, J., Smith, M. K., Ding, G., Chu, J., Wang, H., Li, Q., ... Wang, N. (2013). Drug use and sex work: Competing risk factors for newly acquired HIV in Yunnan, China. *PLoS One, 8*(3), e59050. https://doi.org/10.1371/journal.pone.0059050.

Yadav, G., Saskin, R., Ngugi, E., Kimani, J., Keli, F., Fonck, K., ... Kaul, R. (2005). Associations of sexual risk taking among Kenyan female sex workers after enrollment in an HIV-1 prevention trial. *JAIDS Journal of Acquired Immune Deficiency Syndromes, 38,* 329–334. https://doi.org/10.1097/01.qai.0000166376.23846.38.

Young, A. M., Boyd, C., & Hubbell, A. (2000). Prostitution, drug use, and coping with psychological distress. *Journal of Drug Issues, 30,* 789–800. https://doi.org/10.1177/002204260003000407.

Zhang, C., Li, X., Chen, Y., Hong, Y., Shan, Q., Liu, W., et al. (2014). Alcohol and other drug use, partner violence, and mental health problems among female sex workers in southwest China. *Health Care for Women International, 35,* 60–73. https://doi.org/10.1080/07399332.2012.757317.

Chapter 6
Transitioning Out of Selling Sex

In Chap. 2, we reviewed a variety of factors that motivate women to start selling sex. In this chapter, we review why and how women stop selling sex. Like other topics, this one is not without controversy. The research literature indicates the extent to which women want to transition out of selling sex, and their rationales for doing so, tend to vary depending on their work environments. For example, women who sell sex in street-level contexts often have a negative view of selling sex and are likely to express a desire to transition out of selling sex in the near term. Their transition intentions may be shaped by negative or traumatic experiences. In contrast, some women who sell sex indoors, particularly in high-income countries, view selling sex in either neutral or positive terms (see Chap. 2). These women often envision transitioning out of selling sex at some point, but may express a desire to continue selling sex for the immediate or long-term future. Their transition intentions are more likely to reflect a purposeful personal or professional strategy, rather than strictly a reaction to negative experiences (Ham & Gilmour, 2017).

This chapter explores the many reasons women initiate a transition out of selling sex. We review several conceptual models of the transition process. In addition, we discuss the barriers women may encounter when transitioning out of selling sex and highlight factors that may facilitate successful transitions.

What's in a Name? Exit and Transition Language

In Chap. 1, we noted that the terminology used to describe selling sex (e.g., prostitution, sex work) can sometimes convey the stances people take with regard to this practice and whether it should be supported or limited. To a certain extent, the same is true for the terms used to describe the discontinuation of selling sex.

The term *exit* is often used by programs designed to help women discontinue selling sex. Such programs are more commonly organized by those who favor abolishing

E. Krumrei Mancuso and B. E. Postlethwaite, *Women Who Sell Sex*,
https://doi.org/10.1007/978-3-030-47027-2_6

the sale of sex. Although legalization and sex worker rights activists are certainly not against helping individuals who do not want to sell sex find other means of employment (Ham & Gilmour, 2017), they may take issue with exit language because they believe it implies that selling sex is harmful and perpetuates a negative stigma of those who sell sex (Bowen, 2015; Law, 2013). Further, some have argued that exiting terminology fosters outreach programs premised on the idea that women who sell sex are "naïve, passive victims requiring 'rescue' or 'saving'" (Ham & Gilmour, 2017, p. 749).

To provide a broader context on this terminology, the term *exit* has been widely used in the management and work psychology literatures to describe the phenomenon of an individual who leaves his or her job, often due to dissatisfaction with the work, the employer, or both (e.g., Farrell, 1983; Rusbult, Farrell, Rogers, & Mainous, 1988). Workers who exit do so because they believe the situation is unlikely to improve (Farrell, 1983). Consequently, people who exit their jobs or occupations due to being dissatisfied are unlikely to return.

In this chapter, we use the term *exit* in this broader sense, with the connotation of wishing to permanently discontinue selling sex. We also use *exit* in relation to programs designed, implemented, and labeled as exit programs (e.g., Preble, Praetorius, & Cimino, 2016). Outside of those instances, we use the terminology of *transitioning out* of selling sex because this language may be more inclusive of a broader variety of women's experiences, which can include negative, neutral, or positive reasons for making a change (Bowen, 2015; Law, 2013). For example, rationales for leaving the sex industry range from having a strong negative reaction to the work itself to experiencing positive events such as the achievement of a financial or educational milestone. In addition, transition language has not been associated with the idea of permanence, which is relevant, given that researchers have observed that the commercial sex industry is characterized by mobility. Individuals may move into and out of selling sex, as well as move within the industry itself, such as transferring between brothels or other indoor work venues (e.g., Abel & Fitzgerald, 2012; Bowen, 2015; Gilmour, 2016; Maher, Pickering, & Gerard, 2013; Nixon, Tutty, Downe, Gorkoff, & Ursel, 2002). Finally, the primary reason we favor transition terminology is that it emphasizes that stopping to sell sex is often a complex, multi-step process that unfolds over time rather than a single, discrete event. This parallels movement between occupations that has been described in the careers literature in terms of transition (e.g., Donohue, 2006; Holland, 1997).

Reasons for Initiating a Transition Out of Selling Sex

The empirical literature offers many reasons that women choose to stop selling sex (e.g., Dalla, 2006; Drucker & Nieri, 2018; Gaines et al., 2015; Goldenberg, Engstrom, Rolon, Silverman, & Strathdee, 2013; Ham & Gilmour, 2017; Månsson and Hedin, 1999; Sanders, 2007), which we summarize in Table 6.1. Some of these reasons are about selling sex itself, whereas others are more closely related to external issues

Table 6.1 Reasons for transitioning out of selling sex

Reason category	Push factors	Pull factors
Related to selling sex	• Dissatisfaction with the nature of selling sex • Negative experience with customers • Dissatisfaction with brothel management • Shame about selling sex • Boredom • Personality-job mismatch	• Selling sex was intended to be temporary
Financial	• Low, decreased, or unpredictable earnings • Increased competition	• Achievement of financial objectives • Retirement of debt
Education and alternative work		• Completion of education • Vocational training • Start of an alternate career
Legal	• Increased enforcement of anti-prostitution laws • Harassment by police • Arrest or conviction • Incarceration • Coercive diversion programs	• Supportive diversion programs
Relational	• Escape from an exploitive relationship • Family or friends do not support selling sex • Friends or co-workers have transitioned out of selling sex	• Pregnancy or birth of a child • Desire for monogamy within a relationship • Increased family responsibilities such as child or elder care
Societal	• Stigma • Coercion from social services or other assistance organizations	• Positive support from social services or other assistance organizations
Health and safety	• Risk of violence, or victim of violence • Risk of sexually transmitted infections, or contracting an infection • Major illness • Trauma • Drug or alcohol dependency • Pregnancy • Mental health concerns	• Recovery from physical or mental illness • Professional counseling or therapy • Drug or alcohol treatment
Demographic and other factors	• Age	• Geographic relocation • Spiritual or religious convictions • Planned retirement

such as finances, relationships, or laws. Within each of these categories, we also conceptualize reasons as consisting of push or pull factors. This terminology is more commonly used to describe geographic migration, but we find it useful for understanding the variety of reasons for which women discontinue selling sex and/or transition into other activities.

Push Factors

Push factors consist primarily of factors that women describe as unfavorable, that push them to transition out of selling sex. A review of the literature suggests that push factors tend to be described more often by women who sell sex in street-level contexts than those who sell sex indoors. Women who sell sex on the street often express a desire to stop selling sex to escape violence, drugs, and pimps. Other concerns are about pregnancy and sexually transmitted infections (STIs). Compared to women who work indoors, women selling sex outdoors are more likely to encounter police harassment, arrest, and incarceration, all of which may motivate or necessitate a transition away from selling sex. In some cases, women who face prostitution charges are offered diversion programs in lieu of incarceration. Such programs can be considered push or pull factors, depending on the way in which they are implemented. Wahab and Panichelli (2013) have argued that some of these programs serve the needs of special interests rather than the women themselves, and constitute a form of structural violence against marginalized women. In such instances, these programs may be adverse experiences that push women out of selling sex.

Although the majority of research on transitioning out of selling sex has been conducted among those who sell sex outdoors, recent qualitative research has examined the transition motivations of women who sell sex indoors in brothels, massage parlors, and as independent escorts in high-income countries such as the United States and Australia (e.g., Drucker & Nieri, 2018; Ham & Gilmour, 2017). The push factors described by these women include increased competition, decreased income, poor venue management, and stigma from family members, friends, and society. Age can also become a push factor, if it prevents women from being successful. Conceivably, push factors in these settings can also resemble those of conventional jobs, such as a mismatch between one's personality or interests and the work environment or work itself (e.g., Donohue, 2006; Holland, 1997).

Pull Factors

Pull factors consist primarily of conditions, opportunities, or activities that a woman chooses to pursue instead of selling sex. These are often, but not always, described in favorable or neutral terms, rather than unfavorable terms. Some women describe new or changing relationships as the basis for stopping to sell sex, such as the desire to become sexually monogamous in a personal relationship. Planned retirement is another factor often cited by women discussing their transition intentions. Many women intend to sell sex temporarily and then transition into other things. In a small, qualitative study, British women suggested an ideal retirement age was 30–35 years, although the women expressed mixed feelings about if and when they would in actuality stop selling sex, and many had worked past the ages they had initially set for themselves to stop selling sex (Rickard, 2001). For some women, a change or development in spirituality or religion can underlie the motivation to transition out of selling sex. We classify such motivations as pull factors when the influence of spirituality or religion is uplifting rather than demeaning.

A number of pull factors are described more commonly by women who sell sex in more affluent indoor settings than those who work in street-level contexts. These factors include achieving certain financial goals such as saving for a house, buying a car, or paying off debt. Other women decide to transition out after attending higher education, completing professional training, starting a new job, or establishing their own business. For example, in a study of women selling sex in Australian brothels, Bilardi and colleagues (2011) found that 70% of women would consider transitioning out of selling sex due to finding a better job or starting a business, retiring (56%), or traveling (39%). In this sample, 25% of the women selling sex had looked for a job in the past month and 38% already had jobs outside of selling.

Some women are motivated to transition out of selling sex after coming into contact with professionals or organizations that assist with the exit or transition process (Oselin, 2010). This reason is provided more often by women who work outdoors, because they tend to be more accessible to outreach programs than women who work indoors. We view support services as pull factors when they are empowering rather than coercive, meaning that women have exercised a choice to the use the services and the individuals or organizations providing the services aim to support the women's best interest rather than act out of self-interest. Although some women who sell sex are skeptical of organizations that encourage women to exit, other women indicate they have benefited greatly from support services such as counseling, drug rehabilitation, housing, and vocational training (e.g., Preble et al., 2016). At this point in time, there is little in the way of rigorous, evidence-based evaluations of exit interventions, services, and programs, and researchers have called for more attention to be devoted to this (Preble et al., 2016; Wilson, Critelli, & Rittner, 2015).

A Combination of Factors

Sometimes a woman's desire to transition out of selling sex is influenced by a single push or pull factor, such as being the victim of a serious assault or earning an academic degree. However, it is more common that multiple factors influence a woman's decision in tandem (Oselin, 2010). For example, a woman may be motivated to transition out of selling sex due to safety concerns (a safety push factor) when a friend experiences an assault and quits selling sex (a relational push factor), this motivation is increased by the accumulation of savings that provide economic stability in the absence of selling sex (a financial pull factor), and the transition is facilitated by relocating to another city (a demographic pull factor) to start a new job (an alternative work pull factor).

Conceptual Models of Transition

A number of researchers have organized women's experiences of transitioning out of selling sex into stages or trajectories. Most early work in this regard was based on Ebaugh's (1988) role theory, which focused on how people transition out of any life role through a process of doubt, weighting alternatives, turning points, and establishing an ex-role identity. Since then, a number of conceptual frameworks have been developed specific to transitioning out of selling sex. We will briefly review a number of these models.

In foundational work, Månsson and Hedin (1999) described a life course of selling sex on the basis of their interviews with women who used to sell sex in Sweden. Their model explores a variety of factors that interact together to determine how women transition out of selling sex, including women's internal drives, abilities, and strengths; social networks and relationships; and societal resources and attitudes. They described women breaking away from selling sex in either immediate or gradual fashions, assuming the nature of transitioning out of selling sex would depend largely on the positive or negative critical incidents the women experienced while selling sex and whether the women were loosely involved or ensnared in selling sex.

Building on similar ideas, Sanders (2007) described a trajectory model on the basis of interviews with women who used to sell sex indoors and outdoors in the UK. She described four common forms of transitioning out of selling sex: (1) reactionary routes by which women stop selling sex due to a significant life event, most commonly a violent attack while working, (2) natural progression, based on an accumulation of negative experiences becoming too much for those working outdoors or based on getting older among those working indoors, (3) gradual planning, in which the transition occurs as a result of a conscious plan that unfolds over time, or (4) yo-yoing, when leaving is preceded by frequent movement in and out of selling sex, often as a result of returning to earn money.

Shifting away from the idea of multiple trajectories, Baker, Dalla, and Williamson (2010) developed a stage model for discontinuing to sell sex on the street, with the six stages of (1) immersion in selling sex in which there are no thoughts of leaving, (2) visceral and then conscious awareness of the desire to stop selling sex, (3) deliberate preparation, involving gathering information about formal and informal support for stopping to sell sex, (4) initial exit, when a woman starts to draw on formal and informal support to leave, (5) reentry, in which some women return to selling sex and cycle through previous stages, and (6) final exit, in which a women has made life-encompassing changes with regard to identity, lifestyle, habits, and support sources.

Although a number of these conceptual models take into account re-entry into selling sex, Bowen (2015) criticized exit models for doing so in a way that too narrowly considered selling sex to be pathological and harmful. On the basis of interviews with women currently and formerly selling sex indoors in Canada, Bowen (2015) categorized transitions as encompassing one of three states: (1) sex-work-no-more, where individuals will not return to selling sex, and have often left in order to eliminate harm and gain control in their lives; (2) sex-work-maybe, where individuals have stopped selling sex for specific reasons (such as having a conventional job, being in a romantic relationship, or being concerned about how selling sex will impact mental health or sobriety), but consider selling sex to be an option for the future; and (3) dual-life, where individuals are simultaneously involved in selling sex and conventional work.

These models offer a variety of approaches to understanding the transition out of selling sex from a high-level view. A review of these models highlights three important considerations. First, to be helpful, these models must be flexible enough to accommodate the fact that the nature of a woman's transition out of selling sex is influenced by factors unique to each woman, including intentions, interpersonal relationships, and societal context. Second, the context of selling sex matters. Clear differences have emerged in the transition patterns experienced by women who sell sex in more affluent settings versus street-level contexts. Finally, it is important to understand that transitions out of selling sex are often not final, as reentry is a common phenomenon that must be incorporated into an understanding of the transition process.

Barriers to Transitioning Out of Selling Sex

Some women are content selling sex and intend to keep doing so for the foreseeable future (e.g., Drucker & Nieri, 2018; Ham & Gilmour, 2017). However, for those who desire to transition out of selling sex, it is relevant to consider the barriers they may face. To a certain extent, the barriers to transitioning out of selling sex represent the inverse of the motivational factors by which women first start selling sex (see Chap. 2). That is, the factors that motivate women to start selling sex are often the factors that motivate them to continue rather than discontinue selling sex. As noted in Chap. 1, this book is focused on women who have chosen to sell sex, therefore, this section will not include important barriers associated with overt force, trafficking, and pressure from pimps that keep some women trapped in selling sex.

Månsson and Hedin (1999) offered a three-tiered framework for organizing the barriers that keep women from transitioning out of selling sex that Baker et al. (2010) expanded by adding a fourth tier. Baker et al. (2010, pp. 588–590) provided a useful table summarizing the empirical literature to date that had examined various barriers. We will review this framework and supplement it with a discussion of additional barriers identified in the empirical literature that fit within each tier.

Individual Barriers

The first tier consists of individual factors related to women's internal drives, abilities, interests, dreams, and strategies for adaptation and coping. For example, substance abuse is a prominently studied individual factor. As we explored in more detail in Chap. 5, quantitative and qualitative studies have indicated that substance abuse can be a factor that entrenches women in selling sex (e.g., Gaines et al., 2015; Goldenberg et al., 2013). Other individual factors include additional forms of mental health problems, trauma from childhood, trauma from violence, chronic stress, low self-esteem, feelings of shame or guilt, physical health problems, and lack of knowledge about available social services.

A complex barrier we conceptualize as part of the individual tier is that of identity in both professional and personal forms. Women who have sold sex for an extended period of time may have developed a sense of identity around this activity. Some return to selling sex after transitioning out because they feel it is part of who they are (Nixon, et al., 2002). This can be understood within the context of the professional identity literature, which highlights that professional and personal identity are strongly intertwined and become particularly salient during important life decisions such as a career transition (Ibarra, 1999; Swann, 1987). This explains how, for some women, transitioning out of selling sex may feel like it requires them to abandon how they see themselves, challenging their self-conceptions.

Along similar lines, a barrier some women have described is a sense of internal ambivalence about whether they desire to transition out of selling sex. This occurs when women express the wish to leave, but simultaneously enjoy aspects of selling sex. For example, some women have described that even if they were to transition out of selling sex, they would still keep a few of their customers because they would otherwise miss seeing them (Rickard, 2001).

Finally, some of the structural factors identified by Månsson and Hedin (1999) and Baker et al. (2010) may have individual-level counterparts. For example, access to education is a structural factor, but specific job skills, educational ability, and aptitude for economic self-sufficiency can also be influenced by women's internal drives, abilities, and knowledge. Similarly, although many financial barriers to transitioning out of selling sex are structural in nature, some financial barriers relate to individual desires. While some women need money for basic necessities, others may want money to support luxuries, which can be an individually imposed barrier to transitioning out of selling sex (Drucker & Nieri, 2018; Nixon et al., 2002).

Relational Barriers

The second tier consists of relational factors involving personal relationships and social networks. Previous models have focused on relational factors such as a lack of formal and informal support, strained family relationships, and social isolation.

However, the opposite aspect may also apply in that a significant barrier in stopping to sell sex can be the fear of giving up the social circle women have acquired while selling sex, which may be more supportive and influential than their preexisting relationships (Murphy, 2010). Some women start selling sex without the experience of strong relational and social support in their personal histories. People they encounter while selling sex may make up their first experience of a supportive community. Women may find their relationships with others who share similar life experiences while selling sex to be more genuine than their relationships with outsiders. Interestingly, some women may also feel a sense of obligation to keep selling sex because of their regular customers, with whom they have developed pleasant relationships. Women have expressed a sense of commitment and guilt that keep them from leaving these customers behind (Murphy, 2010).

At the same time, humiliating or denigrating treatment in women's work or private lives can also form a barrier to leaving, primarily because they incite feelings of inferiority and helplessness that may make women feel they are incapable of another way of life (e.g., Wong, Holroyd, & Bingham, 2011).

Finally, many women lack knowledge about transitioning out of selling sex because they lack role models for doing so. Women have reported they either see others fail in their attempts to transition out of selling, or they lose touch with those who successfully transition out and create new lives and social circles for themselves (Rickard, 2001). This means those who remain have little insight or social modeling regarding what it looks like to permanently discontinue selling sex.

Structural Barriers

Månsson and Hedin's (1999) third tier consists of structural factors and societal circumstances, including material conditions, societal resources, public attitudes, and social discourse. Baker et al. (2010) separated into a separate tier what they termed "societal" barriers (discrimination and stigma) from the other structural barriers.

Structural factors include economic conditions, inadequate social services, having a criminal record, and financial barriers. Women who are motivated to start selling sex out of financial necessity are likely to view money as the primary barrier to transitioning out of selling sex (e.g., Brown et al. 2006). This includes needing money for basic living expenses such as food and housing, not being able to find alternative employment due to being homeless or lacking education and job skills, or a scarcity of employment opportunities in the local economy (e.g., Bowen, Canfield, Trostle, & Harley, 2015; Goldenberg et al., 2013; Hankel, Heil, Dewey, & Martinez, 2016; Nixon et al., 2002). In some cases, alternative work is available but pays considerably less, making it less desirable (e.g., Drucker & Nieri, 2018; Ham & Gilmour, 2017). This is particularly the case for women without higher education or specialized job training.

Some women have identified a lack of relevant social services, such as effective drug treatment or psychological help, as barriers in their attempts to stop selling sex (e.g., Rickard, 2001). At times the barriers women face are imposed by the institutions and social structures designed to help. For example, a study of injection drug using women who sold sex in Mexico indicated that experiencing a greater police presence and reporting money extortion by police were both associated with a lower likelihood of stopping to sell sex (Gaines et al., 2015). Further, Brown et al. (2006) have provided examples of women selling sex in the inner-city in Canada who faced stigma from social assistance staff and were denied social benefits to which they were entitled. These factors can make it difficult for women who would like to stop selling sex to transition successfully.

Finally, important structural or societal barriers include social perceptions of women who sell sex. This includes the experience of stigma and discrimination. Learmonth, Hakala, and Keller (2015) powerfully illustrated such barriers with focus group accounts of black women selling sex on the street in South Africa. They found that gendered experiences intersected with oppression related to class and race to produce a uniquely disempowered position that served as a barrier to exit for these women.

Interacting Barriers

The roadblocks to exiting may become particularly strong when multiple barriers interact with each other. This often occurs across boundaries of the framework tiers. For example, stigma, a structural/societal barrier, can contribute to fear of rejection in relationships, a relational barrier. Societal stigma can also result in internalized stigma, an individual factor, by which women come to experience shame, self-disgust, guilt, and regret. These feelings may contribute to the belief that selling sex is the only work one is worthy of doing. Thereby, shame and selling sex can perpetuate one another in a cyclical fashion, causing women to be trapped by their own judgments of themselves. In this way, internalized stigma is associated with feelings of helplessness and inevitability regarding selling sex (Wong et al., 2011).

Another example of interacting barriers was provided by Brown et al. (2006), who described how women selling sex in the inner-city in Canada faced stigma from social assistance staff, were denied social benefits to which they were entitled, and were made to feel uncomfortable by social workers. These represent societal barriers of social stigma and discrimination; however, they also represent relational barriers of being isolated within one's community and other structural barriers of economic hardship and a lack of opportunity to be supported by social services. This illustrates how women can experience a multi-layering of barriers that compound one another to make a transition out of selling sex all the more difficult.

Successful Transitions Out of Selling Sex

Having reviewed the many barriers women can face in transitioning out of selling sex highlights how remarkable a successful transition is. As noted, a transition out of selling sex need not necessarily be permanent for a woman to view it as successful, given that a minority of women may stop selling sex for a particular reason, but consider selling sex to be a viable option again in the future (Bowen, 2015). Therefore, we define a successful transitions out of selling sex as one in which a woman discontinues selling sex for the period of time desired, which may be permanently, and does not reenter the sex trade against her deeper desires or better judgment. As described, women tend to lack knowledge and modeling of successful transitions out of selling sex, because those who go before them often enter new social circles and discontinue previous relationships. Research can help fill this need by offering insight into the factors that contribute to successful transitions, which can be used to provide psychoeducation to those who would like to pursue such a life change.

As a first step in this direction, Cimino (2012) applied the integrative model of behavioral prediction to understanding successful exit from selling sex on the street. This theory focuses on accounting for the role of agency, societal contexts, environmental constraints, and personality traits in the exit process in a systematic way. According to this model, intentions to discontinue selling sex will be a function of a person's attitudes, norms, self-efficacy, and belief system. A successful transition is likely to occur if a woman has strong intentions to exit, has the necessary skills and abilities to exit, and does not experience environmental constraints that prevent her from exiting. Cimino (2012) argued that this model offers a testable theory for predicting a successful exit from selling sex on the street. However, to date there has not been a rigorous empirical investigation of the model.

Studies that follow women's transitions out of selling sex over time are rare and limited in generalizability due to the specificity of the samples employed. However, they provide the best insights to date about what factors may account for the difference between successful and unsuccessful attempts to transition out of selling sex and they are able to evaluate quit-re-entry patterns over time. A number of studies have followed women with substance addictions over time. Gaines and colleagues (2015) followed a sample for one year consisting of 467 injection drug using women in an HIV prevention program who sold sex in Mexico. The program was not focused on transitioning out of selling sex, but the researchers were able to evaluate a number of factors associated with successful initial cessation of selling sex. These included a number of the push and pull factors we explored that motivate women to stop selling sex, specifically: having income from sources other than selling sex, having increased access to health services, receiving substance abuse treatment, having financial dependents to care for, and having experienced sexual abuse by the police. Similar studies in the United States have echoed the importance of psychosocial services. For example, a national study of women receiving substance abuse treatment, of which 533 women sold sex, indicated that receiving more extensive substance abuse treatment and receiving more mental health and social services were associated with a greater likelihood of having transitioned out of selling sex one year later (Burnette, Schneider, Timko, & Ilgen, 2009). Unfortunately, these studies did not extend beyond a one-year period.

Additional insights can be gained from Dalla (2006), who followed up with a sample of women who sold sex on the street, three years after initial interviews. Although attrition was high (58%) and only a sample of 18 women was attained at follow-up, this is one of the few studies that offers a longer-term comparison between women who successfully and unsuccessfully attempted to stop selling sex. Although these themes are likely not generalizable due to the small size and unique characteristics of the sample, a number of differences were observed between those who were and weren't successful in transitioning out of selling sex along the themes of relationships, personal initiative, work attitudes, religion, and mental health.

With regard to relationships, a key difference was found in the women's informal social networks. Those who were successful in exiting tended to cut ties with previous acquaintances, whereas those who were not successful in exiting maintained a social circle of individuals involved in selling sex and drug trafficking. As may be intuitive, research has observed positive associations between having a greater number of friends who use drugs and trading sex for money or drugs (e.g., Edwards, Halpern, & Wechsberg, 2006). This illustrates the importance of peer social norms in influencing behavior with regard to selling sex.

Nearly all of the women in Dalla's (2006) study (89%) had been involved with formal support agencies in their attempts to transition out of selling sex, however, those who were successful also displayed personal initiative in obtaining knowledge, internalizing information, and applying new tools in their lives. Those who were not successful described either a lack of commitment to making necessary changes or described an expectation that others were responsible for fixing their life situations. Thus, having an internal locus of control and exerting personal initiative seemed to be key to a successful transition out of selling sex. Similarly, those who were successful at transitioning out viewed other forms of employment as an opportunity to obtain skills and demonstrate competence, whereas those who returned to selling sex were more focused on short-term financial gain and expressed a lack of patience and commitment when it came to conventional employment, which researchers have noted often involves work characterized by low pay, poor working conditions, and little opportunity for advancement (e.g., Drucker & Nieri, 2018; Ham & Gilmour, 2017).

Finally, two factors seemed to differentiate the two groups almost completely. First, religion, spirituality, or God were described as important by all of those whose transitions out of selling sex were successful, but only by 15% of those whose transitions were unsuccessful. It seems religion may have provided a source of renewal and strength for those who were able to create different lives for themselves. Second, over half of those who were unsuccessful in their attempts to transition away from selling sex raised the topic of mental health concerns, whereas this was not brought up by any of those who successfully transitioned out of selling sex. This seems to indicate that those who were not able to break with selling sex may have faced more barriers with regard to mental health.

Discussion

This chapter has explored a variety of topics related to transitioning out of selling sex, including factors that motivate women to initiate a transition, factors that are associated with successful transition, and factors that may impede successful transitions. What is missing from this chapter is a clear discussion of the *outcomes* of transitioning out of selling sex. That is, how do women fare once they have transitioned out of selling sex, and how does their wellbeing compare to that while selling sex or before selling sex? Unfortunately, there is little empirical evidence to speak to these questions given the limited amount of longitudinal research that has been conducted on transitioning out of selling sex. The one exception to this is work that has been conducted among substance users. Research has indicated that women with substance abuse problems experience better mental health and substance use outcomes when they stop selling sex (e.g., Burnette, Schneider, Timko, & Ilgen, 2009). Thus, it seems clear that some women will benefit from transitioning out of selling sex. However, more research is needed to examine the outcomes of transitioning out of selling sex for a fuller range of women who sell sex.

To date, the majority of research on transitioning out of selling sex has examined women in their natural trajectories. Therefore, the available findings cannot necessarily directly be applied to intervention efforts on behalf of helping professionals. However, the literature reveals many variables that would be useful to explore more systematically in future research as potential points of intervention for aiding women who wish to transition out of selling sex. The common puzzle pieces that seem relevant to a beneficial, multifaceted approach include mental health and substance abuse treatment, social services, and ways to support financial stability. In Text Box 6.1, we explore the idea of microfinance and entrepreneurship training programs to address the financial needs of women who desire to transition out of selling sex. In some locations, structural interventions may also be necessary to address exploitative policing practices or discriminative practices among social services. Although the empirical evidence is limited, we offer some initial questions for consideration on the basis of current themes in the literature that may be useful to helping professionals working with women transitioning out of selling sex (see Table 6.2). We explore more detailed treatment themes for clinicians working with women transitioning out of selling sex in Chap. 7.

Table 6.2 Initial questions for consideration in working with women transitioning out of selling sex

- Has the woman expressed an intent to transition out of selling sex? What push and pull factors are informing her decision?
- What individual, relational, or structural barriers does the woman face? Does the woman experience a multi-layering of barriers? Do the barriers interact with or compound one another?
- Does the woman have a substance abuse problem or mental health concern that needs immediate attention?
- What practical needs must be addressed as part of the transition (housing, childcare, finances, etc.)?
- Has the woman tried to transition out of selling in the past? To what extent was this successful? If not successful, why not?
- Has the woman had contact with exit or other support organizations? What was the nature and quality of this contact? Is she interested in future contact with such organizations?
- What alternative employment opportunities are available? Do any require vocational or other training?
- What relational and social resources are available for support in transitioning out? Is this support short-term or long-term?

Text Box 6.1 Microfinance and Entrepreneurship Training Programs as Aids to Transition

As noted in this chapter, financial issues often serve as a significant barrier to transitioning out of selling sex. These issues can be complex and difficult to address. Women who wish to stop selling sex need to replace their income derived from selling sex but may encounter a lack of suitable alternative employment opportunities in their local area. The barriers to transitioning are even greater when women lack the education or job skills necessary to secure one of the work opportunities that exists in their communities. Under circumstances such as these, microfinance initiatives and entrepreneurial training programs that enable women to start their own business ventures may be valuable aids to the transition process. Some women are drawn to selling sex because they view it as an entrepreneurial pursuit. Given this, some women who wish to stop selling sex may find entrepreneurial opportunities quite attractive. New ventures offer a potential for flexibility and control that is unmatched by most other forms of work. Although some women selling sex may never have considered the possibility of starting their own business, in several of the studies we reviewed, women from high-income countries identified saving enough money to start a business as either a goal for selling sex, or a reason for stopping once the goal was achieved (e.g., Bilardi et al., 2011; Ham & Gilmour, 2017).

Microfinance

Microfinance involves providing small loans to aid in the startup or growth of a small business venture (for a review, see Brau & Woller, 2004). Loans typically range from the local equivalent of a few hundred to a few thousand dollars, with repeat borrowers having access to increasingly more capital after they successfully repay smaller value loans. Most typically, microfinance loans are made by nonprofit or non-governmental organizations that specialize in this type of lending; however, loans can also be made by traditional financial institutions or governments. Microfinance initiatives often have explicit social goals attached, such as reducing poverty, empowering disenfranchised individuals and groups (frequently women), and reducing income inequality. Interest in microfinance has grown significantly over the past several decades. In 2006, the Nobel Peace Prize was jointly awarded to Mohammed Yunus and the Grameen Bank, the microfinance institution he founded, for his pioneering work promoting microlending to the poor in Bangladesh.

Microfinance institutions do not just provide loans, rather the organizations deliver a suite of coordinated services to increase the likelihood that the borrower's venture is successful and the loan is repaid. High impact programs incorporate a number of features such as frequent contact between lenders and borrowers (sometimes weekly), financial literacy education, vocational or entrepreneurial skills training, and the creation of peer support groups to encourage accountability. These unique features serve to reduce the number of loan defaults while increasing program impact. However, it is quite costly to deliver a high level of services to inexperienced borrowers. As a result, microfinance loans typically carry a high interest rate. Further, there is debate with regard to the actual impact that microfinance has on poverty. For example, research in Bangladesh has shown that microfinance helps both loan recipients (particularly women) and their local communities (Khandker, 2005), while research in Sub-Saharan Africa has shown that microfinance can have positive impacts, but can also do harm (Van Rooyen, Stewart, & De Wet, 2012).

Organizations involved in supporting women who wish to stop selling sex can consider microfinance as a potential adjunct to their existing service offerings. Microlending could be provided directly by the support organization, or it could be delivered by a partner microfinance organization with the necessary knowledge, staff, and expertise. Given the cost and complexity involved in providing very small loans, support organizations who are new to this area may have greater success by partnering with an established microfinance organization.

Entrepreneurial Skills Training, Coaching, and Mentoring

Microfinancing may not be appropriate for women who have sold sex and managed to save enough money to launch their own new ventures. Nevertheless, many of these women would benefit from specialized training, coaching, and mentoring to develop their entrepreneurial skills as well as a viable business plan. Although some may argue that entrepreneurs are born rather than made, specific business skills can certainly be taught.

Transition support organizations may lack the human or financial resources to deliver entrepreneurial programming and support themselves. This presents an excellent opportunity for support organizations to partner with successful entrepreneurs and business schools in their communities. Many entrepreneurs and business owners are willing to share their expertise, as are many retired managers and executives. Likewise, business schools often seek ways for their students and faculty to move beyond the classroom and use their business knowledge to positively impact their communities and society as a whole. For example, one of the primary global business school accreditors, the Association to Advance Collegiate Schools of Business (AACSB), has identified Engagement and Societal Impact as one of the new proposed standards for 2020 (AACSB, 2020). Providing entrepreneurial skills training to women seeking to transition out of selling sex would certainly contribute toward this goal.

Case Study: An Entrepreneurial Program for Young Women Selling Sex in Rwanda

Programme Communautaire de Lutte contre le SIDA (PCLS) is a community AIDS control program providing comprehensive services to women selling sex in Byumba, a city in northern Rwanda. Hakizimana, Ntezimana, and Uwingenzi (2018) examined the group's efforts to improve the lives of young women (ages not specified) selling sex by developing a multi-faceted intervention program that included entrepreneurial skills training as well as other support services. Prior to participating in the program, the 57 young women sampled had experienced high rates of physical (93%), economic (79%), sexual (72%), and psychological (65%) violence. They also reported struggling with poverty (75%), trauma (72%), STIs (58%), economic dependence (53%), and feelings of depression and isolation (46%).

The women received entrepreneurial skills training in addition to having access to advocacy, counseling, legal assistance, drug abuse prevention education, and assistance with health insurance. Entrepreneurial skills training included regular meetings, peer education, presentations, and focus group discussions. After participating in the program, 63% of women had become members of group savings and loan associations, 44% had joined local women's organizations, 23% had joined human rights and domestic/gender based violence organizations, 21% had joined community volunteer associations, and 20% had joined HIV/AIDS clubs. Thus, participation in skills training appears to have empowered women to engage with multiple aspects of their community. After participating, a third of the sample (33%) were engaged in small business activities. In addition, the women reported engaging in a number of agricultural activities such as buying cattle (47%), purchasing livestock (37%), or investing in other agricultural activities (32%). These agricultural investments were viewed by the local official in charge of social affairs as being an optimal savings strategy, because "animals are viewed as savings banks, since the livestock represent significant capital that can be easily and quickly converted into money or food in times of need" (Hakizimana et al., 2018, p. 20).

Women participating in the program demonstrated a number of other positive economic outcomes. All of the women reported having bank accounts after starting their businesses. Likewise, all of the participants reported being able to pay for their own health insurance, 86% reported renting business or residential property, and 26% reported paying for vocational training school fees. Finally, all of the women stated that their lives had changed as a result of participating in the program, and, overall, participants reported a 75% reduction in selling sex and poverty (these measures were reported together).

Not all microfinance or entrepreneurship training programs will see this level of success. However, this unique case from Rwanda illustrates the positive impacts that are possible when microfinance and entrepreneurial skills trainings are integrated into a holistic transition support program. Regardless of location, financial issues are a central factor in determining whether women who want to stop selling sex will be able to do so. Programs that seek to help women transition away from selling sex must keep women's financial barriers in mind when designing and delivering services. Microfinance and entrepreneurship training are but two tools among others (such as financial literacy, career guidance, job search, and vocational training) that can be considered when aiding women in overcoming their financial barriers.

Finally, it is important to consider the spirit within which services are provided to women transitioning out of selling sex. Our experience is that those whose goal it is to help women transition out of selling sex can be guided by a variety of attitudes that dictate the nature and quality of their approach. It is useful for social service and other helping organizations not only to be thoughtful about their end goals with regard to working with women who desire to transition out of selling sex, but also to examine their ideologies about who these women are. Viewing these women as passive, weak, or incompetent, or seeing a victim rather than a whole person, may all covertly encourage approaches that are not beneficial, whether taking the form of subtle stigmatization, discrimination or coercion, or overt abuse and exploitation. Such approaches can spiral into cultures that are demeaning and dehumanizing to women who sell sex. We have seen in the literature that stigma, coercion, and violence can be push factors that motivate women to discontinue selling sex, but they can also form barriers to successfully transitioning out of selling sex. More importantly, such approaches can be harmful to the women involved. If the goal is to care for the wellbeing of women in addition to helping them meet their goals of successfully transitioning out of selling sex, this calls for approaches grounded in a holistic view of the women, including respect for their autonomy. It seems that the most helpful approaches focus on encouragement, empowerment, and capitalizing on malleable pull factors to help women transition into preferred activities in life.

References

AACSB. (2020, February 3). *2020 guiding principles and standards for business accreditation (Draft 2)*. Tampa, FL: AACSB.

Abel, G. M., & Fitzgerald, L. J. (2012). 'The street's got its advantages': Movement between sectors of the sex industry in a decriminalised environment. *Health, Risk & Society, 14*, 7–23. https://doi.org/10.1080/13698575.2011.640664.

Baker, L. M., Dalla, R. L., & Williamson, C. (2010). Exiting prostitution: An integrated model. *Violence Against Women, 16*, 579–600. https://doi.org/10.1177/1077801210367643.

Bilardi, J. E., Miller, A., Hocking, J. S., Keogh, L., Cummings, R., Chen, M. Y., et al. (2011). The job satisfaction of female sex workers working in licensed brothels in Victoria, Australia. *Journal of Sexual Medicine, 8*, 116–122. https://doi.org/10.1111/j.1743-6109.2010.01967.x.

Bowen, R. R. (2015). Squaring up: Experiences of transition from off-street sex work to square work and duality—concurrent involvement in both—in Vancouver, BC. *Canadian Review of Sociology, 52,* 429–449. https://doi.org/10.1111/cars.12085.

Bowen, E. A., Canfield, J. P., Trostle, A., & Harley, D. (2015). Predictors of stable housing for homeless women leaving a sex-work program. *Families in Society, 96,* 268–276. https://doi.org/10.1606/1044-3894.2015.96.36.

Brau, J. C., & Woller, G. M. (2004). Microfinance: A comprehensive review of the existing literature. *Journal of Entrepreneurial Finance, 1*(9), 1–28.

Brown, J., Higgitt, N., Miller, C., Wingert, S., Williams, M., & Morrissette, L. (2006). Challenges faced by women working in the inner city sex trade. *Canadian Journal of Urban Research, 15,* 36–53.

Burnette, M. L., Schneider, R., Timko, C., & Ilgen, M. A. (2009). Impact of substance-use disorder treatment on women involved in prostitution: Substance use, mental health, and prostitution one year after treatment. *Journal of Studies on Alcohol & Drugs, 70,* 32–40. https://doi.org/10.15288/jsad.2009.70.32.

Cimino, A. N. (2012). A predictive theory of intentions to exit street-level prostitution. *Violence Against Women, 18,* 1235–1252. https://doi.org/10.1177/1077801212465153.

Dalla, R. L. (2006). "You can't hustle all your life": An exploratory investigation of the exit process among street-level prostituted women. *Psychology of Women Quarterly, 30,* 276–290. https://doi.org/10.1111/j.1471-6402.2006.00296.x.

Donohue, R. (2006). Person-environment congruence in relation to career change and career persistence. *Journal of Vocational Behavior, 68,* 504–515. https://doi.org/10.1016/j.jvb.2005.11.002.

Drucker, J., & Nieri, T. (2018). Female online sex workers' perceptions of exit from sex work. *Deviant Behavior, 39,* 1–19. https://doi.org/10.1080/01639625.2016.1257890.

Ebaugh, H. R. F. (1988). *Becoming an ex: The process of role exit*. Chicago: University of Chicago Press.

Edwards, J. M., Halpern, C. T., & Wechsberg, W. M. (2006). Correlates of exchanging sex for drugs or money among women who use crack cocaine. *AIDS Education and Prevention, 18,* 420–429. https://doi.org/10.1521/aeap.2006.18.5.420.

Farrell, D. (1983). Exit, voice, loyalty, and neglect as responses to job dissatisfaction: A multidimensional scaling study. *Academy of Management Journal, 26,* 596–607. https://doi.org/10.5465/255909.

Gaines, T. L., Urada, L. A., Martinez, G., Goldenberg, S. M., Rangel, G., Reed, E., … Strathdee, S. A. (2015). Short-term cessation of sex work and injection drug use: Evidence from a recurrent event survival analysis. *Addictive Behaviors, 45,* 63–69. https://doi.org/10.1016/j.addbeh.2015.01.020.

Gilmour, F. E. (2016). Work conditions and job mobility in the Australian indoor sex industry. *Sociological Research Online, 21*(4). https://doi.org/10.5153/sro.4166.

Goldenberg, S. M., Engstrom, D., Rolon, M. L., Silverman, J. G., & Strathdee, S. A. (2013). Sex workers perspectives on strategies to reduce sexual exploitation and HIV risk: A qualitative study in Tijuana, Mexico. *PLoS One, 8*(8). https://doi.org/10.1371/journal.pone.0072982.

Hakizimana, L., Ntezimana, A., & Uwingenzi, M. (2018). Entrepreneurship as a key to anthropo-social and economic development in Rwanda: Case of young female sex workers assisted by PCLS in Byumba City, Byumba Sector in Gicumbi District (2016–2017). *International Journal of Research in Sociology and Anthropology, 4*(1), 16–23. https://doi.org/10.20431/2454-8677.0401003.

Ham, J., & Gilmour, F. (2017). 'We all have one': Exit plans as professional strategy in sex work. *Work, Employment & Society, 31,* 748–763. https://doi.org/10.1177/0950017016666198.

Hankel, J., Heil, M., Dewey, S., & Martinez, N. (2016). Characteristics of women seeking services at a transitional housing facility for women leaving street-based sex work: Implications for social service providers. *Journal of Social Service Research, 42,* 41–56. https://doi.org/10.1080/01488376.2015.1077188.

Holland, J. L. (1997). *Making vocational choices: A theory of vocational personalities and work environments* (3rd ed.). Englewood Cliffs, NJ: Prentice Hall.

Ibarra, H. (1999). Provisional selves: Experimenting with image and identity in professional adaptation. *Administrative Science Quarterly, 44,* 764–791.

Khandker, S. R. (2005). Microfinance and poverty: Evidence using panel data from Bangladesh. *World Bank Economic Review, 19,* 263–286. https://doi.org/10.1093/wber/lhi008.

Law, T. (2013). Transitioning out of sex work: Exploring sex workers' experiences and perspectives. In E. van der Muelen, E. M. Durisin, & V. Love (Eds.), *Selling sex: Experience, advocacy, and research on sex work in Canada* (pp. 101–110). Toronto: UBC Press.

Learmonth, D., Hakala, S., & Keller, M. (2015). "I can't carry on like this": Barriers to exiting the street-based sex trade in South Africa. *Health Psychology and Behavioral Medicine, 3,* 348–365. https://doi.org/10.1080/21642850.2015.1095098.

Maher, J., Pickering, S., & Gerard, A. (2013). *Sex work: Labour, mobility, and sexual services.* London: Routledge.

Månsson, S. A., & Hedin, U.-C. (1999). Breaking the Matthew effect—On women leaving prostitution. *International Journal of Social Welfare, 8,* 67–77. https://doi.org/10.1111/1468-2397.00063.

Murphy, L. (2010). Understanding the social and economic contexts surrounding women engaged in street-level prostitution. *Issues in Mental Health Nursing, 31,* 775–784. https://doi.org/10.3109/01612840.2010.524345.

Nixon, K., Tutty, L., Downe, P., Gorkoff, K., & Ursel, J. (2002). The everyday occurrence: Violence in the lives of girls exploited through prostitution. *Violence Against Women, 8,* 1016–1043*f*. https://doi.org/10.1177/107780120200800902.

Oselin, S. S. (2010). Weighing the consequences of a deviant career: Factors leading to an exit from prostitution. *Sociological Perspectives, 53,* 527–549. https://doi.org/10.1525/sop.2010.53.4.527.

Preble, K. M., Praetorius, R. T., & Cimino, A. (2016). Supportive exits: A best practices report for a sex worker intervention. *Journal of Human Behavior in the Social Environment, 26,* 162–178. https://doi.org/10.1080/10911359.2015.1082852.

Rickard, W. (2001). 'Been there, seen it, done it, I've got the t-shirt': British sex worker's reflect on jobs, hopes, the future and retirement. *Feminist Review, 67,* 111–132. https://doi.org/10.1080/0141778015.

Rusbult, C. E., Farrell, D., Rogers, G., & Mainous, A. G., III. (1988). Impact of exchange variables on exit, voice, loyalty, and neglect: An integrative model of responses to declining hob status satisfaction. *Academy of Management Journal, 31,* 599–627. https://doi.org/10.2307/256461.

Sanders, T. (2007). Becoming an ex-sex worker: Making transitions out of a deviant career. *Feminist Criminology, 2,* 74–95. https://doi.org/10.1177/1557085106294845.

Swann, W. B., Jr. (1987). Identity negotiation: Where two roads meet. *Journal of Personality and Social Psychology, 6,* 1038–1051. https://doi.org/10.1037/0022-3514.53.6.1038.

Van Rooyen, C., Stewart, R., & De Wet, T. (2012). The impact of microfinance in Sub-Saharan Africa: A systematic review of the evidence. *World Development, 40,* 2249–2262. https://doi.org/10.1016/j.worlddev.2012.03.012.

Wahab, S., & Panichelli, M. (2013). Ethical and human rights issues in coercive interventions with sex workers. *Affilia: Journal of Women and Social Work, 28,* 344–349. https://doi.org/10.1177/0886109913505043.

Wilson, B., Critelli, F. M., & Rittner, B. A. (2015). Transnational responses to commercial sexual exploitation: A comprehensive review of interventions. *Women's Studies International Forum, 48,* 71–80. https://doi.org/10.1016/j.wsif.2014.10.005.

Wong, W. W., Holroyd, E., & Bingham, A. (2011). Stigma and sex work from the perspective of female sex workers in Hong Kong. *Sociology of Health & Illness, 33*(1), 50–65. https://doi.org/10.1111/j.1467-9566.2010.01276.x.

Chapter 7
Clinical Considerations for Mental Health Professionals Working with Women Who Sell Sex

The previous chapters of this book have explored a variety of psychological concepts relevant to women who choose to sell sex. In this chapter, we review implications for mental health professionals. This chapter is written with psychotherapists in mind, however, other helping professionals may glean insights as they see fit. To date, very little has been written about providing competent care to psychotherapy clients who are or have been involved in sex work. Given the paucity of clinical writings, the goal of this chapter is to explore therapeutic themes that may be relevant to women who sell sex and seek mental health services. However, future research will be required to evaluate the effectiveness of particular interventions among this population. Further, this chapter is not intended to suggest that all women who sell sex face particular psychological problems. Clinical assessment will indicate which of the discussed themes, if any, are relevant to the treatment of a particular psychotherapy client.

We begin with some basic and ethical considerations for working with women who sell sex. Next, the chapter focuses on a variety of themes relevant to individualizing treatment, including suggestions for assessment and therapeutic work with women who sell sex, women transitioning out of selling sex, and women who no longer sell sex.

Basic Considerations

Competent Care

Clinicians desiring to work with women who sell sex should first evaluate their knowledge and experience in working with this population, and when necessary, seek education, consultation, or supervision. Education is necessary to move beyond simplistic understandings of women who sell sex and to avoid misconceptions that get

E. Krumrei Mancuso and B. E. Postlethwaite, *Women Who Sell Sex*,
https://doi.org/10.1007/978-3-030-47027-2_7

in the way of providing appropriate care (Shaver, Lewis, & Maticka-Tyndale, 2011). Educational resources may be helpful in promoting an understanding of women who sell sex as heterogeneous, with diverse needs.

Clinicians should be aware, as noted throughout this book, that the research literature on selling sex is most abundant in the study of the most visible and easily accessible women, which in many countries tends to be those engaged in street prostitution, those incarcerated, those in substance abuse or crisis treatment programs, and those receiving social services. This means the available research on mental health among women who sell sex is most informative with regard to women who have the most visible life challenges and psychological and social problems. Thus far, much less is known about the experiences and mental health of women who sell sex legally, who work in certain indoor settings, or who work as elite escorts. Much more clinically oriented research and writing specific to working with women who sell sex is needed. Despite the limitations of the literature, incorporating the available research and clinical writings into therapeutic work will ensure that practices are as current, evidence-based, and effective as possible.

Therapist Self-awareness

A first step in providing competent care to women who sell sex, is for clinicians to evaluate their comfort levels in providing such treatment. Selling sex is a topic that people tend to have strong feelings about, and clinicians are not immune to this. It is natural for clinicians to bring their personal perspectives and biases into the therapy room. Personal instincts and values can be a benefit for guiding the course of treatment. However, personal beliefs and biases can also become problematic, particularly when a therapist lacks awareness about these personal viewpoints and how they are impacting treatment. Denying one's perspectives can result in harm to psychotherapy clients, such as coercing or marginalizing psychotherapy clients unknowingly. Awareness, on the other hand, helps therapists guard against biases getting in the way of competent care. Clinicians who are new to working with women who sell sex may increase self-awareness through exercises such as journaling, identifying and exploring assumptions, identifying and exploring emotions, noticing physical tension, and considering countertransference issues. Owning one's values and viewpoints is the first step in shifting them from a treatment liability to an asset.

Hopefully it goes without saying that psychotherapy clients must be treated with respect and care. This includes sensitivity to the challenges and barriers psychotherapy clients face as well as respect for the autonomy of psychotherapy clients and their choices. Clinicians who realize they cannot fully respect psychotherapy clients as persons of value due to involvement in sex work will best serve such individuals by referring them to another competent clinician.

Informed Consent

Self-awareness can be thought of as discovering and owning one's viewpoints as a therapist. The next step is informed consent, which involves sharing these viewpoints with psychotherapy clients and explaining how they inform the therapeutic work. Beyond a general informed consent process typical of therapy, clinicians working with women who sell sex should educate potential psychotherapy clients about their own views on selling sex as well as their goals for treatment. This is no different than other areas of clinical work where clinicians may have strong personal feelings about the goals of therapy. For example, a marriage therapist should inform psychotherapy clients if he or she plans to fight for their marriage or advocate for the individual desires or mutual goals of those in the relationship. Similarly, a clinician working with religious issues should inform psychotherapy clients if he or she views religion as helpful or harmful in the psychotherapy client's life (or both), and in what ways. Some clinicians will believe that selling sex is harmful and that it's always in a woman's best interest to discontinue; others may want to advocate for a woman's choice to sell sex and celebrate it as respectable way to earn a living. Whatever the case may be, clinicians should explain their perspective in an understandable way, so that psychotherapy clients can make an informed choice about whether the professional is a good fit for them and the type of help they are seeking.

A Multifaceted and Integrated Approach

Consideration should be given to the fact that some women who sell sex may not have the financial means, transportation, or even willingness to identify themselves in order to seek mental health services. Finding ways to provide mental health services in settings and modalities that these women are more likely to access would be of great benefit to them. One option is to move toward greater integration of mental and physical health services, for example, in community health centers. Technology can also be a resource in providing some forms of mental health care to women who have concerns about anonymity.

Providing mental health care to women who sell sex will often be most effective when it is coordinated alongside assistance from other professionals. Clinicians can assess the need for referrals to healthcare, social services, or substance abuse treatment. In addition, women who sell sex may benefit greatly from peer networking and social support systems. Helping to facilitate such social connections can be crucial given that some women who sell sex lacked healthy forms of social support to begin with, or may have created distance in their social relationships to keep their choice to sell sex a secret. They are also likely to have encountered social stigma. These circumstances can contribute to social isolation, which is often detrimental to wellbeing. Alternatively, some women who sell sex are involved in maladaptive networks that negatively influence decision-making and encourage risky behaviors (e.g., Murphy, 2010). Working to create caring social relationships and networks can be a challenging but essential task for women who sell sex.

Individualized Care

One of the most important themes in this book has been the great variety among women who sell sex and their diversity of experiences. This makes it difficult to provide any kind of absolutes about providing mental health care for this population, other than that assessment and treatment must be individualized. In reality, it is misleading to even think of this group as one population. Even though we encourage clinicians to incorporate the available literature on women who sell sex into their clinical work, it is important to not fall into the myth of sameness, by assuming that every woman who sells sex will have had similar experiences, exhibit the same characteristics, or present with the same clinical issues. A one-size-fits-all approach will simply not work. The subsequent sections of this chapter explore how to create an individualized framework for providing care to women who sell sex and themes that may be relevant to various stages of transition in and out of selling sex.

Therapist Self-care

Before shifting to the topic of individualized care, a final basic consideration is that therapists' self-care is important for those working with women who sell sex. This is true for a number of reasons. As reviewed in Chap. 3, many women who sell sex experience physical and sexual violence, particularly in street-level contexts. Research has indicated that in some settings, providing care to women who sell sex can result in vicarious traumatization (Brady, Guy, Poelstra, & Brokaw, 1999; Jung, Song, Chong, Seo, & Chae, 2008; Schauben & Frazier, 1995). Particularly, having a higher case load of psychotherapy clients who have experienced sexual violence and more exposure to sexual abuse content in sessions is associated with more symptoms of trauma and PTSD among helping professionals, even independent of the professionals' own histories of victimization. For these reasons, it is important for clinicians working with women who sell sex to possess healthy coping and self-care mechanisms, particularly if a substantial portion of the case load at any given time involves processing sexual violence.

Another important theme is that clinicians working with women who sell sex can experience courtesy stigma (Phillips, Benoit, Hallgrmsdottir, & Vallance, 2012). Courtesy stigma occurs by association with a stigmatized individual or group, when a stigmatized individuals' *spoiled identity* becomes associated with another party (Goffman, 1963). Limited work has indicated that the stigma of sex work can transfer to others such as researchers or helping professionals (Phillips et al., 2012). It is important for clinicians to use self-care mechanisms to cope with the potential stressors of courtesy stigma, in order to promote their own mental health and wellbeing, as well as to prevent courtesy stigma from becoming a barrier to providing care to women who sell sex.

Providing Individualized Care Within a Lifecycle Framework of Selling Sex

Developmental models have been applied to many aspects of life, including work. For example, Donald Super applied a life-span, life-space approach to understanding career development, identifying that people go through different stages in relation to work that are impacted by context (e.g., Super, 1990, 1992). Although we do not intend to apply Super's model to selling sex as a career, there are some useful insights that can be distilled from his theory and applied to the phenomenon of selling sex, including that a woman's experience in relation to selling sex may develop and change over time in key ways. As such, the implication for helping professionals are quite different depending on whether a woman is actively involved in selling sex, in the process of transitioning out of selling sex, or no longer selling sex. We will consider implications for clinical work within each of these stages.

Working With Women Who Sell Sex

Most mental health services surrounding the sale of sex are geared toward women who are in the process of exiting or have already exited. However, those who are actively selling sex are equally in need of competent mental health services. This includes women who desire to transition out, women who desire to sell sex as long as possible, and women who feel ambivalent about exiting.

It is useful for clinicians to develop an understanding of an individual woman's experience with selling sex and how this relates, if at all, to her clinical presentation. This includes gaining a basic understanding of whether or not, how, or to what extent:

- selling sex relates to the psychotherapy client's treatment goals
- the psychotherapy client is satisfied with her choice to sell sex
- selling sex leads to benefits and/or harm to the psychotherapy client and her loved ones
- the psychotherapy client's wellbeing is impacted by selling sex
- the psychotherapy client is self-aware about the impact of selling sex on her life and identity
- the psychotherapy client's motivations to sell sex are internally and/or externally based
- selling sex is related to the psychotherapy client's life goals
- the psychotherapy client leads an integrated life or compartmentalizes selling sex
- the psychotherapy client experiences harmony, friction, or risk with regard to selling sex in relation to physical, emotional, psychological, relational, spiritual, and/or religious domains of life.

In gathering a picture of the psychotherapy client, clinicians should keep in mind that, although selling sex will influence a woman's experiences, many other factors will influence her experiences as well, including her gender, culture, socioeconomic status, and idiosyncratic characteristics. Further, it is important to realize that selling sex and demographic and multicultural factors can mutually influence each other (e.g., Clarke, Clarke, Roe-Sepowitz, & Fey, 2012). Therefore, treatment planning must take into account the experience of selling sex, personal, demographic, and multicultural factors, and how they interact with one another.

Table 7.1 provides suggestions for topics that may be relevant to cover in an intake interview with a psychotherapy client who sells sex. These questions are meant to be tailored to the therapeutic conversation in a flexible way in which the clinician focuses only on those topics that seem relevant to a particular psychotherapy client. To be clear, these questions should supplement standard intake questions so that a clinician does not overlook relevant clinical concerns by focusing on selling sex to the neglect of other issues.

Following a thorough assessment, treatment should be tailored to the individual needs and goals of a psychotherapy client. Next, we briefly discuss a number of themes that may be relevant to therapeutic work with women who sell sex. Detailed discussion of the associated treatments is beyond the scope of this brief introduction.

Table 7.1 Intake questions for women who sell sex—supplement to standard intake questions

History of selling sex

1. When was the first time you remember thinking about selling sex?
2. How did you first become involved in selling sex? How old were you?
3. Was another person or other people involved in your selling sex?
4. What are all the forms of sex work you have been involved in? What types of settings have you worked in?
5. How has selling sex changed your life for the better? How has it changed your life for the worse?
6. Have you ever stopped selling sex for a period of time or tried to stop for a period of time? What was this like?

Present factors surrounding selling sex

1. Why are you currently involved in selling sex? In what settings do you work?
2. To what degree do you enjoy selling sex? Does it provide you with meaning? Fulfillment? Confidence? Social connection?
3. To what extent is selling sex a source of difficulty in your life? Does it cause you feelings of guilt? Shame? Anger? Confusion? Doubt? Anxiety? Fear? Stress? Insignificance? Isolation from others?
4. Have you experienced physical/sexual violence while selling sex? If so, from whom? How have these experiences impacted you?
5. Are there times that you don't feel safe when selling sex?
6. Do you view selling sex as relevant to your reasons for seeking therapy?

Future with regard to selling sex

1. Would you like to continue selling sex? If so, for how long?
2. How does selling sex relate to your life goals?
3. Do you ever have mixed thoughts or feelings about selling sex? Describe them.
4. Have you thought about quitting selling sex? If so, what stopped you?

Social experience

1. Who knows that you sell sex? How did important relations respond when they found out?
2. Are there people who don't know that you sell sex, but you wish they knew ? Describe these relationships.
3. Where do you turn for social support? Describe your closest relationships.
4. Who is supportive of you selling sex? Who is not supportive of you selling sex?
5. Have you experienced social stigma or discrimination for selling sex? If so, describe.

Sexuality

1. How was sexuality expressed in your environment when you grew up?
2. How did you first express your sexuality?
3. How have your views of sexuality changed over the course of your life?
4. What has helped nurture your sexuality? What has been damaging to your sexuality?
5. How do you currently view yourself as a sexual being? Does this relate to selling sex?

Work experiences

1. Is selling sex your primary source of income?
2. If you are involved in other work, does this coordinate well or poorly with selling sex?

Personal characteristics in relation to selling sex

1. How important is your gender identity to you? Does it relate to your experience of selling sex?
2. How important is your racial or ethnic identity to you? Does it relate to your experience of selling sex?
3. How much education do you have? Does this relate to your choice to sell sex?
4. Are you a religious or spiritual person? Does this relate to your experience of selling sex?

Exploration of Views of the Body and Sexuality

Views of the body and sexuality come from a myriad of sources, including family of origin, peers, education system, media, culture, and religion. For some women, dissonance between their conscious or unconscious beliefs about their bodies or sexuality in relation to the activity of selling sex can result in difficult emotions, such as guilt, shame, anger, or confusion, or in mental health symptoms, such as depression or anxiety. When relevant, treatment can focus on uncovering a psychotherapy client's beliefs about her body and sexuality and exploring the sources of these beliefs. To minimize dissonance, women can evaluate the beliefs they hold and make more conscious choices about which values and beliefs to affirm and live by, and which values and beliefs may warrant change. As a case example, Text Box 7.1 explores the theme of how religion relates to views of the body and sex, with potential implications for women who sell sex.

Text Box 7.1 Links Between Religion and Views of the Body and Sexuality

Historically, religion has played a large role in determining sexual values and behaviors across cultures. Religious views of sex have ranged widely in nature, including religiously imposed sexual restrictions, sex as a form of worship (including sacred/temple prostitution), sexuality as an ultimate expression of the divine, and sex as a gift from God to be expressed within specific relational confines. Although not frequently studied, there is no reason to believe that women who sell sex do not possess religious beliefs or backgrounds that influence the way they experience the activity of selling sex.

Some contemporary research has examined specific links between religion and views of the body and sexuality, by exploring concepts such as sanctification and desecration. Although this research has been conducted primarily among Christian samples within the general population, and not specifically among women selling sex, the findings offer some food for thought.

A number of studies have shown that sanctifying one's body, meaning believing that one's body is holy or sacred, is associated with more body appreciation and satisfaction, more health-promoting and health-protective behaviors, a greater experience of unity with the body, less body objectification and depersonalization, and greater awareness of the body (Jacobson, Hall, & Anderson, 2013; Jacobson, Hall, Anderson, & Willingham, 2016; Mahoney et al., 2005). On the other hand, viewing one's body as corrupt or separate from one's sense of personhood is associated with less body appreciation and more body shame (Jacobson et al., 2016).

Although exploratory in nature, examining in psychotherapy whether women who sell sex perceive their bodies in sacred or corrupt terms may offer a foundation for understanding their motivations and responses to selling sex.

For example, a lack of sanctification or viewing one's body as corrupt may be associated with more risk-taking behaviors when selling sex. The links may be bi-directional as well, as selling sex could result in experiencing a separation between one's body and one's sense of self, as previous qualitative work has indicated, resulting in less body appreciation and more body shame.

A related line of research has indicated that religious beliefs about sex can influence sexual behaviors and sexual satisfaction. Specifically, those who view sex as sacred within marriage or non-marital loving relationships engage in sex more frequently within those contexts and experience more sexual satisfaction (Hernandez-Kane & Mahoney, 2018; Murray-Swank, Pargament, & Mahoney, 2005).

The concepts of sacred loss and desecration lie opposite to sanctification. They involve the perception that something considered sacred or holy has been lost or violated. Although these concepts have rarely been studied in relation to the body or sex, a number of studies in other domains have identified that suffering the loss or violation of something sacred is associated with more negative affect, physical health symptoms, poorer mental health including anxiety and depression, and interestingly, also more personal and spiritual growth (see Pargament & Mahoney, 2005, for review). The effects of sacred loss and desecration are not attributable to merely viewing something as a negative event; the findings persist even when controlling people's perceived negativity of an experience.

On these bases, it may be worthwhile to explore clinically whether women who sell sex attach any sacred attributes to sex within their personal relationships, or even within the context of selling sex, and if so, how that influences their experiences. Previous research suggests that those who view sex as sacred within marital or loving relationships might experience selling sex as a loss or violation of the sacred. In such cases, the consequences can include a host of difficult emotional, physical, and mental health symptoms that can be addressed in treatment. Interestingly, previous research suggests that such experiences can also form the foundation of personal and spiritual growth, which can be explored in therapy as well.

Exploration of Self-concept

A theme from Super's career development model that can be adapted to working with women who sell sex is exploration of the role of self-concept in relation to selling sex. Super argued that people base their work decisions on their self-attributes and beliefs about their abilities. Clinicians may explore if and how selling sex is a manifestation of selfhood and whether the woman experiences a match between her self-concept and her experience with selling sex. This may include an exploration of the woman's views of her abilities, traits, and values.

Exploration of Strengths

Much of the research and writing about women who sell sex has focused on barriers, limitations, and problems. It is essential for successful treatment to also explore, emphasize, and build on women's strengths. This includes reinforcing psychological resilience, building positive coping and self-care mechanisms, and focusing on opportunities for positive emotions and personal growth. Consistent with the broaden-and-build theory of positive emotions (Fredrickson, 2001), emphasizing such strengths can broaden psychotherapy clients' physical, intellectual, social, and psychological resources. This can even help build trait resilience, a personal characteristic that helps one recover from adversity, setbacks, and crises (Fredrickson, Tugade, Waugh, & Larkin, 2003).

Exploration of Life Roles and Social Context

A second theme from Super's career development model that can be adapted to working with women who sell sex involves the multiple social roles of a woman in relation to selling sex. Super believed that work unfolds in the context of all life roles of an individual. Selling sex cannot fully be grasped without taking into account a woman's whole constellation of life roles. How the woman's various central life roles impact one another is key to wellbeing and life satisfaction. Of particular interest to clinical work is when selling sex is a core life role that conflicts with other salient life roles that make up the woman's identity, such as being a citizen, homemaker, student, employee, daughter, sister, and/or parent.

It is relevant for clinicians to explore these themes with an understanding of the social stigma faced by women who sell sex (see Chap. 3). Clinical work may focus on how well selling sex fits within the psychotherapy client's social context, including whether her environment is accepting or hostile to her choice. Relevant themes include the extent to which the psychotherapy client experiences social support, social conflict, and social isolation on the basis of selling sex.

Trauma Work

The research reviewed in this book indicates that women who sell sex often report high lifetime incidence of abuse and tend to experience physical and sexual violence and victimization at rates higher than the general population (see Chap. 3). This is particularly true for women working in street-level contexts. Some research has indicated that PTSD symptoms increase proportionally to the number of years women have sold sex (Jung et al., 2008). Some women who sell sex consider violence from customers to be a more concerning work hazard than the health-related risks associated with sexually transmitted infections, because violence is less predictable and more prevalent (Sanders, 2004). Other than customers, perpetrators of violence can include pimps, other women who sell sex, police, intimate partners, and the general public. Outside of the experience of violence, clinicians can also explore with psychotherapy clients whether selling sex, itself, has been experienced as traumatic.

Assertiveness Training

Women who sell sex must negotiate the conditions of their transactions, including the nature of sex acts, the time limit, the amount of payment, and the use of protection. Those who are not able to assert themselves in these matters may expose themselves to dangers and health risks. Not all women who sell sex work in safe, secure, or financially independent conditions that enable them to successfully exert control (e.g., Gysels, Pool, & Nnalusiba, 2002). However, for those who are in positions to negotiate the conditions of their work, assertiveness training can be a useful harm-reduction tool.

Treatment of Mood Disorders

The research reviewed in this book indicates that depression and anxiety are prevalent among many samples of women who sell sex and often at higher rates than in the general population (see Chap. 4). Some qualitative research has suggested that women who sell sex consider the emotional and psychological consequences of selling sex to be more concerning than the risk of violence from customers or the health-related risks of selling sex (Sanders, 2004). Further, some research has indicated that depressive symptoms among women who sell sex are associated with engaging in more behaviors that place the women at risk for HIV infection (Alegría et al., 1994). Thus, mood disorders are not only concerning for their own sake, but also because they can interfere with the motivation to engage in behaviors that reduce physical health risks. Additionally, mood disorders may increase isolation among women who sell sex, thereby reducing social support and help seeking. For these reasons, it is important to screen for anxiety and depression among women who sell sex.

Substance Abuse Treatment

As reviewed in Chap. 5, there are substantial links between selling sex and substance use and abuse, most strongly in street-level contexts. Substance abuse treatment can be tailored to relevant themes that have been highlighted in the literature, including addressing co-morbid mental health concerns and specific risks for relapse. For example, under the self-medication hypothesis, women who rely on alcohol or substances to cope with traumas associated with selling sex should simultaneously be engaged in trauma work and taught alternative coping skills. In addition, a common consideration in substance abuse treatment is the establishment of supportive relationships and communities that are substance free in an effort to minimize triggers for alcohol and drug use. This is of particular importance to women who sell sex, given that the secrecy surrounding their work can be isolating and limit them to social connections with others who are heavily involved in alcohol and substances, especially when this is an expectation within the work setting (e.g., some brothels and clubs). Therefore, involvement in support groups and (re)establishing healthy social networks can be very valuable aspects of treatment.

For some women, selling sex, itself, is a barrier to alcohol or substance abuse recovery efforts. Research has indicated that among women who sell sex and have substance abuse problems, those who continue to sell sex exhibit poorer substance-related outcomes than those who discontinue (Burnette, Schneider, Timko, & Ilgen, 2009). In this research, discontinuing selling sex was associated with less substance use, higher rates of abstinence, and fewer mental health symptoms.

Motivational Interviewing

For women who feel ambivalent about selling sex, motivational interviewing can be used to explore whether they would like to make a life change, and if so, provide them the motivation for doing so. Motivational interviewing originated with work on problematic drinking and addictive behaviors (Miller, 1983; Miller & Rollnick, 1991), but has been applied widely to behavior change. Extensive clinical writings exist on the topic. In short, motivational interviewing is used to help psychotherapy clients explore and resolve ambivalence about life decisions. It is directive, in the sense that clinicians help psychotherapy clients consider making changes by exploring discrepancies between their current behaviors and their ideal behaviors or life goals. At the same time, the approach is fully supportive of the psychotherapy client and her self-efficacy. The belief is that the psychotherapy client is responsible for choosing and carrying out any life change. The next section provides more detailed information about treatment themes for those who decide they would like to transition out of selling sex.

Working with Women Transitioning Out of Selling Sex

In Chap. 6, we explored research themes relevant to women transitioning out of selling sex. Insights from Chap. 6—such as the understanding that ceasing to sell sex is a process and insight into the various stages that can be part of this process—will likely be helpful to clinicians tailoring assessment and intervention efforts to the specific needs of psychotherapy clients. The needs of women exiting sex trade can be thought of as existing on practical and psychological levels.

Practical Level

Practical needs will be the greatest for women actively transitioning out of selling sex in comparison to psychotherapy clients who continue to sell sex or no longer sell sex. Women who desire to stop selling sex may need help planning their transitions to be successful (Sanders, 2007). Although research comparing women who have and haven't been successful in transitioning out is rare, the available data suggest that common needs in the initial stages of exit can include safety, housing, separation from previous friends and acquaintances, and substance abuse treatment (Dalla, 2006). Screening for these initial needs is essential, as addressing these needs will allow women to pursue other logistical goals, such as job skills training or securing alternative employment.

Subsequently, it is crucial to address potential social needs. Women who sell sex often distance themselves from personal relationships to keep choice to sell sex private and they may narrow their social circle to others who work in the sex industry. Many accounts indicate that women who have stopped selling sex struggle to broaden their social circles and make new friends, but that doing so is essential for success (e.g., Brown et al., 2006; Hedin & Månsson, 2004). Psychotherapy clients may need support as they integrate into new communities and develop or repair relationships and networks. This may mean connecting with local community organizations such as community centers, churches, or participating in neighborhood events. Some psychotherapy clients will also need time to foster or restore healthy emotional attachments with family members.

At this stage, some women may also need to be connected with legal resources for reconciling with separated children, such as services that advocate for women who have had child protective agencies involved. They may also benefit from parent training, parenting support, and information about childcare.

In sum, in the early stages, services that provide logistical help may be key in supporting women whose goal it is to transition out of selling sex. Clinicians can play a role by helping women identify and connect with a broad range of resources.

Psychological Level

Although it is important to support the practical needs of the transition, clinical work will focus primarily on addressing psychological needs. Women have indicated in interviews that the period immediately after discontinuing to sell sex is a very difficult time (Månsson & Hedin, 1999) and that it can be difficult for women to obtain mental health care due to a general lack of knowledge about selling sex in the mental health field (Hedin & Månsson, 2004). To this end, clinicians will benefit from understanding the conceptual stage models reviewed in Chap. 6.

During the transition period, treatment will likely focus primarily on stabilization. Mental health assessment should include a focus on the common challenges that occur for women who have recently stopped selling sex. This may include treating crisis reactions involving acute anxiety (Månsson & Hedin, 1999). Motivational interviewing may also be key in helping women shift to a place of initiative in the midst of a potentially overwhelming life change. Once any present crisis reactions subside, work can shift toward the themes discussed in the next section.

Working with Women Who No Longer Sell Sex

Women with a history of selling sex are as diverse as women who currently sell sex. Some will have exited the sex trade under substantial distress whereas others may have retired after a relatively happy career. Women with a history of selling sex who seek treatment may benefit from working on the themes already discussed for women actively selling sex. For example, the effects of trauma, comorbid mood disorders, or substance abuse problems will not magically cease upon exiting the sex trade. It can be useful to explore themes that may underlie or exacerbate mental health concerns, such as particular views of the body, sexuality, and self-concept. Equally, focusing on strengths, resilience, and resources will be crucial to wellbeing and a fulfilling life for women who no longer sell sex. The current section supplements the themes already discussed for women actively selling sex, with consideration of additional themes that may be relevant among women who no longer sell sex.

Developing a New Self-narrative

Women who have recently stopped selling sex may need to cognitively come to terms with their experience of selling sex. Some women will grapple to understand the role of sex trade in their lives and why they became involved. Some will experience heavy feelings of shame, guilt, and regret. Shame may be the result of a deep-seated conflict between one's views of self or sexuality and one's experience selling sex. Shame may also represent an internalized sense of self-contempt stemming from condemning attitudes experienced from others. Many researchers have documented the negative reactions women who sell sex have experienced from those around them, ranging from avoidance to serious acts of discrimination (e.g., Brown et al., 2006; Månsson & Hedin, 1999). Those who have recently exited may continue to face a sense of marginalization outside of their familiar world of selling sex. These circumstances can deeply influence women's views of themselves.

Women who struggle with self-defeating life narratives may benefit from narrative therapy. This approach is useful in helping women overcome problem-saturated stories about themselves that have been shaped by dominant cultural narratives that objectify and dehumanize marginalized groups, including those who sell sex. The goal is to help women re-author their guiding life story in a way that is based on thick (comprehensive, rich, multifaceted) rather than thin (superficial, one-dimensional, stereotypical) descriptions of themselves. This relates to the next theme of identity work.

Exploring Themes of Personal and Professional Identity

Hayne and Shepherd (2011) have examined career transitions following traumatic life events. They recounted the experience of a Marine who was injured in Iraq and subsequently left military service. Prior to his traumatic injury, he would always introduce himself by saying, "Hi, I'm Aaron; I'm a Marine" (p. 501). Hayne and Shepherd (2011) argued that his career as a Marine was the foundation of his self-narrative, the story he told himself about who he was and where he belonged. After his injury he stopped introducing himself because he "didn't know what to say" (p. 501). Aaron's career was his source of identity and losing it left him questioning who he was.

Unlike Aaron, women who sell sex are not likely to lead with this fact in their introductions. However, like Aaron, women who have sold sex for an extended period of time are likely to have developed a strong identity revolving around the sale of sex. Not surprisingly, work identity and personal identity are often strongly intertwined. Issues of identity can be particularly salient following important life decisions, such as transitioning out of selling sex (Ibarra, 1999; Swann, 1987). For some women, breaking with selling sex requires abandoning their previous identity. This may leave a void, particularly for women whose identities revolved exclusively around selling sex, ultimately requiring them to question or change their self-conceptions. In such cases, exploring self-concept can be a helpful step. Therapeutic work can include focusing on psychotherapy clients' potential future selves, careers, and roles rather than on the past. They may also benefit from support as they face vulnerability and self-consciousness in the process of forging a new identity.

As noted in Chap. 6, viewing selling sex as part of one's identity can be a factor in returning to selling sex after exiting. Therefore, those who desire to remain out of the sex trade, yet continue to struggle with the transition to a new life and identity, may benefit from ongoing maintenance therapy to identify and address the triggers for reentering the sex trade.

Psychoeducation Surrounding Sexuality

In addition to exploring views of the body and sex as discussed above, women who no longer sell sex may benefit from some forms of psychoeducation about sexuality. Although some women may experience a sense of sexual self-esteem and confidence from selling sex that translates into their personal lives, many women who have sold sex describe grappling with their personal sense of sexuality (Bellhouse, Crebbin, Fairley, & Bilardi, 2015). Some research has indicated that the majority of women find sex in their personal lives to be less enjoyable once they start selling sex (Kramer, 2004). It is a common phenomenon for women to mentally separate sex with customers from sex in their personal lives (e.g., Oerton & Phoenix, 2001; Sanders, 2002). This often involves a variety of protective mechanisms, such as screening bodily experiences and arousal during sex with customers (Bernstein, 2007; Sanders, 2005). When such protective mechanisms transfer into women's personal lives, psychoeducation can be a useful tool to help psychotherapy clients understand how to let go of these habits during sex in their personal lives. Where relevant, clinical attention may also focus on healing from sexual violence or trauma encountered while selling sex.

Discussion

In Chap. 3, we discussed the serious social stigma that many women who sell sex encounter on a regular basis. Such stigma can form a barrier to women who sell sex seeking mental health care (Rayson & Alba, 2019; Zehnder, Mutschler, Rössler, Rufer, & Rüsch, 2019). A wealth of research has shown that individuals who suffer from mental health concerns also encounter significant stigma because of their mental health status and this stigma can also obstruct care seeking and treatment participation (Corrigan, 2004). Thus, women who sell sex and have mental health concerns face compounding stigmas that may detract from their ability to pursue care. Given these considerable barriers to reaching out for help, clinicians might consider it an honor and privilege to have trust bestowed in them by a woman who sells sex or has sold sex in the past.

When women who sell sex seek mental health services, their presenting concerns may or may not be directly linked with selling sex. In this chapter, we have identified some basic considerations that may be of use to therapists who work with women who sell sex or have sold sex in the past. These include the importance of competent care, therapist self-awareness, and informed consent. Furthermore, psychological care will be most effective when it is integrated into a holistic package of assistance that addresses financial, social, and physical health needs.

Therapists must understand that women who sell sex are a heterogeneous group—one woman's experience selling sex may vary markedly from another's, even if their situations appear similar. This calls for an individualized approach to evaluation and treatment. In this chapter, we made use of a lifecycle framework as a tool for thinking about how to develop an individualized treatment approach. That is, the type of psychological care that is appropriate will depend, in part, on whether a psychotherapy client is actively selling sex, is transitioning out of selling sex, or is no longer selling sex. Clinical assessment will help determine which, if any, of the treatment themes discussed in this chapter are relevant to a particular psychotherapy client.

References

Alegría, M., Vera, M., Freeman, D. H., Robles, R., Santos, M. C., & Rivera, C. L. (1994). HIV infection, risk behaviors, and depressive symptoms among Puerto Rican sex workers. *American Journal of Public Health, 84,* 2000–2002. https://doi.org/10.2105/AJPH.84.12.2000.

Bellhouse, C., Crebbin, S., Fairley, C. K., & Bilardi, J. E. (2015). The impact of sex work on women's personal romantic relationships and the mental separation of their work and personal lives: A mixed-methods study. *PLoS One, 10*(10), e0141575. https://doi.org/10.1371/journal.pone.0141575.

Bernstein, E. (2007). Sex work for the middle classes. *Sexualities, 10,* 473–488. https://doi.org/10.1177/1363460707080984.

Brady, J. L., Guy, J. D., Poelstra, P. L., & Brokaw, B. F. (1999). Vicarious traumatization, spirituality, and the treatment of sexual abuse survivors: A national survey of women psychotherapists. *Professional Psychology: Research and Practice, 30,* 386–393. https://doi.org/10.1037/0735-7028.30.4.386.

Brown, J., Higgitt, N., Miller, C., Wingert, S., Williams, M., & Morrissette, L. (2006). Challenges faced by women working in the inner city sex trade. *Canadian Journal of Urban Research, 15,* 36–53.

Burnette, M. L., Schneider, R., Timko, C., & Ilgen, M. A. (2009). Impact of substance-use disorder treatment on women involved in prostitution: Substance use, mental health, and prostitution one year after treatment. *Journal of Studies On Alcohol & Drugs, 70,* 32–40. https://doi.org/10.15288/jsad.2009.70.32.

Clarke, R. J., Clarke, E. A., Roe-Sepowitz, D., & Fey, R. (2012). Age at entry into prostitution: Relationship to drug use, race, suicide, education level, childhood abuse, and family experiences. *Journal of Human Behavior in the Social Environment, 22,* 270–289. https://doi.org/10.1080/10911359.2012.655583.

Corrigan, P. (2004). How stigma interferes with mental health care. *American Psychologist, 59,* 614–625. https://doi.org/10.1037/0003-066x.59.7.614.

Dalla, R. L. (2006). "You can't hustle all your life": An exploratory investigation of the exit process among street-level prostituted women. *Psychology of Women Quarterly, 30,* 276–290. https://doi.org/10.1111/j.1471-6402.2006.00296.x.

Fredrickson, B. L. (2001). The role of positive emotions in positive psychology: The broaden-and-build theory of positive emotions. *American Psychologist, 56,* 218–226. https://doi.org/10.1037/0003-066X.56.3.218.

Fredrickson, B. L., Tugade, M. M., Waugh, C. E., & Larkin, G. R. (2003). What good are positive emotions in crises? A prospective study of resilience and emotions following the terrorist attacks on the United States on September 11th, 2001. *Journal of Personality and Social Psychology, 84,* 365–376. https://doi.org/10.1037/0022-3514.84.2.365.

Goffman, E. (1963). *Stigma: Notes on the management of spoiled identity*. Englewood Cliffs, NJ: Prentice-Hall.

Gysels, M., Pool, R., & Nnalusiba, B. (2002). Women who sell sex in a Ugandan trading town: Life histories, survival strategies and risk. *Social Science and Medicine, 54,* 179–192. https://doi.org/10.1016/S0277-9536(01)00027-2.

Hayne, J. M., & Shepherd, D. (2011). Toward a theory of discontinuous career transition: Investigating career transitions necessitate by traumatic life events. *Journal of Applied Psychology, 96,* 501–524. https://doi.org/10.1037/a002145.

Hedin, U. C., & Månsson, S. A. (2004). The importance of supportive relationships among women leaving prostitution. *Journal of Trauma Practice, 2,* 223–237. https://doi.org/10.1300/j189v02n03_13.

Hernandez-Kane, K. M., & Mahoney, A. (2018). Sex through a sacred lens: Longitudinal effects of sanctification of marital sexuality. *Journal of Family Psychology, 32*(4), 425–434. https://doi.org/10.1037/fam0000392.

Ibarra, H. (1999). Provisional selves: Experimenting with image and identity in professional adaptation. *Administrative Science Quarterly, 44,* 764–791.

Jacobson, H. L., Hall, M. E. L., & Anderson, T. L. (2013). Theology and the body: Sanctification and bodily experiences. *Psychology of Religion and Spirituality, 5*(1), 41–50. https://doi.org/10.1037/a0028042.

Jacobson, H. L., Hall, M. E. L., Anderson, T. L., & Willingham, M. M. (2016). Temple or prison: Religious beliefs and attitudes toward the body. *Journal of Religion and Health, 55*(6), 2154–2173. https://doi.org/10.1007/s10943-016-0266-z.

Jung, Y.-E., Song, J.-M., Chong, J., Seo, H.-J., & Chae, J.-H. (2008). Symptoms of posttraumatic stress disorder and mental health in women who escaped prostitution and helping activists in shelters. *Yonsei Medical Journal, 49,* 372–382. https://doi.org/10.3349/ymj.2008.49.3.372.

Kramer, L. A. (2004). Emotional experiences of performing prostitution. *Journal of Trauma Practice, 2*(3/4), 187–197. https://doi.org/10.1300/j189v02n03_10

Mahoney, A., Carels, R. A., Pargament, K. I., Wachholtz, A., Leeper, L. E., Kaplar, M., & Frutchey, R. (2005). The sanctification of the body and behavioral health patterns of college students. *International Journal for the Psychology of Religion, 15*(3), 221–238. https://doi.org/10.1207/s15327582ijpr1503_3.

Månsson, S. A., & Hedin, U. C. (1999). Breaking the Matthew effect—On women leaving prostitution. *International Journal of Social Welfare, 8,* 67–77. https://doi.org/10.1111/1468-2397.00063.

Miller, W. R. (1983). Motivational interviewing with problem drinkers. *Behavioural Psychotherapy, 11,* 147–172. https://doi.org/10.1017/S0141347300006583.

Miller, W. R., & Rollnick, S. (1991). *Motivational interviewing: Preparing people to change addictive behavior*. New York: Guilford.

Murphy, L. (2010). Understanding the social and economic contexts surrounding women engaged in street-level prostitution. *Issues in Mental Health Nursing, 31,* 775–784. https://doi.org/10.3109/01612840.2010.524345.

Murray-Swank, N. A., Pargament, K. I., & Mahoney, A. (2005). At the crossroads of sexuality and spirituality: The sanctification of sex by college students. *International Journal for the Psychology of Religion, 15,* 199–219. https://doi.org/10.1207/s15327582ijpr1503_2

Oerton, S., & Phoenix, J. (2001). Sex/bodywork: Discourses and practices. *Sexualities, 4,* 387–412. https://doi.org/10.1177/136346001004004001.

Pargament, K. I., & Mahoney, A. (2005). Sacred matters: Sanctification as a vital topic for the psychology of religion. *International Journal for the Psychology of Religion, 15*(3), 179–198. https://doi.org/10.1207/s15327582ijpr1503_1.

Phillips, R., Benoit, C., Hallgrmsdottir, H., & Vallance, K. (2012). Courtesy stigma: A hidden health concern among front-line service providers to sex workers. *Sociology of Health & Illness, 5,* 681–696. https://doi.org/10.1111/j.1467-9566.2011.01410.x.

Rayson, J., & Alba, B. (2019). Experiences of stigma and discrimination as predictors of mental health help-seeking among sex workers. *Sexual and Relationship Therapy, 34,* 277–289. https://doi.org/10.1080/14681994.2019.1628488.

Sanders, T. (2002). VI. The condom as psychological barrier: Female sex workers and emotional management. *Feminism & Psychology, 12,* 561–566. https://doi.org/10.1177/0959353502012004016.

Sanders, T. (2004). A continuum of risk? The management of health, physical and emotional risks by female sex workers. *Sociology of Health & Illness, 26,* 557–574. https://doi-org.lib.pepperdine.edu/10.1111/j.0141-9889.2004.00405.x.

Sanders, T. (2005). "It's just acting": Sex workers' strategies for capitalizing on sexuality. *Gender, Work and Organization, 12,* 319–342. https://doi.org/10.1111/j.1468-0432.2005.00276.x.

Sanders, T. (2007). Becoming an ex-sex worker: Making transitions out of a deviant career. *Feminist Criminology, 2,* 74–95. https://doi.org/10.1177/1557085106294845.

Schauben, L. J., & Frazier, P. A. (1995). Vicarious trauma: The effects on female counselors of working with sexual violence survivors. *Psychology of Women Quarterly, 19,* 49–64. https://doi.org/10.1111/j.1471-6402.1995.tb00278.x.

Shaver, F. M., Lewis, J., & Maticka-Tyndale, E. (2011). Rising to the challenge: Addressing the concerns of people working in the sex industry. *Canadian Review of Sociology, 48,* 47–65. https://doi.org/10.1111/j.1755-618x.2011.01249.x.

Super, D. E. (1990). A life-span, life-space approach to career development. In D. Brown & L. Brooks (Eds.), *Career choice and development: Applying contemporary theories to practice* (pp. 197–261). San Francisco, CA, US: Jossey-Bass.

Super, D. E. (1992). Toward a comprehensive theory of career development. In D. H. Montross, C. J. Shinkman, D. H. Montross, & C. J. Shinkman (Eds.), *Career development: Theory and practice* (pp. 35–64). Springfield, IL, England: Charles C Thomas, Publisher.

Swann, W. B., Jr. (1987). Identity negotiation: Where two roads meet. *Journal of Personality and Social Psychology, 6,* 1038–1051. https://doi.org/10.1037/0022-3514.53.6.1038

Zehnder, M., Mutschler, J., Rössler, W., Rufer, M., & Rüsch, N. (2019). Stigma as a barrier to mental health service use among female sex workers in Switzerland. *Frontiers in Psychiatry, 10,* 32. https://doi.org/10.3389/fpsyt.2019.00032.

Chapter 8
Putting It All Together: Themes in the Psychological Research on Women Who Sell Sex

This book has provided a review of research on psychological topics conducted among women who sell sex, including research on the motivations for selling sex, sources of stress, mental health concerns, and themes in transitioning out of selling sex. We also discussed the clinical implications of this research for mental health providers. In this final chapter, we highlight some of the key points of the book, beginning with the idea that selling sex is a complex, multi-faceted phenomenon, which makes it problematic to broadly generalize about the psychological motivations, experiences, and outcomes of women who sell sex. We then address the important question of whether selling sex is psychologically harmful to women. We acknowledge the limitations of our review and the existing literature and identify areas where there is both opportunity and need for additional research. We conclude with a call for researchers, mental health practitioners, and policymakers to use psychology both to further our understanding of sexual commerce and to ultimately improve the welfare of women for whom this is a relevant topic.

The Multi-faceted Nature of Selling Sex

If anything is clear from this book, it is that selling sex is a complex and multi-faceted phenomenon. This makes it challenging to draw general conclusions about selling sex. Rather than describing women who sell sex as a diverse group, it may be more appropriate to acknowledge that they are not really a group at all, but rather individuals among whom some have more in common than others. Women who sell sex represent many different ages, races, ethnicities, socio-economic statuses, sexual orientations, educational levels, religious faiths, backgrounds, personal dispositions, life skills, life experiences, and lifestyles. In addition, the conditions, relationships, routines, works schedules, and types of services offered when it comes to commercial sex differ. Weitzer (2010) used the *polymorphous paradigm* to describe that selling

E. Krumrei Mancuso and B. E. Postlethwaite, *Women Who Sell Sex*,
https://doi.org/10.1007/978-3-030-47027-2_8

sex isn't uniform, but rather is "a constellation of occupational arrangements, power relations, and worker experiences" characterized by "substantial variation" (p. 6). Our review suggests that this diversity applies to the psychology of selling sex, as well.

In Chap. 2, we discussed how women are motivated to sell sex for a variety of reasons, ranging from financial need and substance abuse to personal interest and rational choice. The research is clear that in some settings, women choose selling sex over other employment opportunities available to them. The choice to sell sex, like any life decision, is influenced by women's life experiences and conditions. Women who sell sex are often motivated not by one single influence, but by multiple factors. As in other areas of psychology, single-factor causal models are not to be found. Along these lines, it is important to consider base rates in any discussion of the precursors of selling sex. For example, while the prevalence of childhood abuse seems to be higher among samples of women who sell sex than among the general population, this clearly does not mean that all, or even the majority, of individuals who experience childhood abuse will sell sex. In one of the few available prospective research designs, Widom and Kuhns (1996) found that approximately 9% of their participants with a history of childhood abuse and neglect ended up selling sex by early adulthood, in comparison to 3% of the control participants who had not experienced abuse and neglect. This means that those who experienced childhood abuse or neglect were three times more likely to sell sex. Although a three-fold difference between the groups is substantial, this should not overshadow the fact that less than one in 10 of the participants who were abused as children ended up selling sex.

In Chap. 3, we discussed the social context of selling sex. Our review indicates that women's experiences of selling sex seem to range from extremely traumatic to quite positive in nature. This range of experiences appears, in part, to result from the diversity of environments in which women sell sex. Selling sex can be stressful due to the threat of violence, concerns over the legal status of sexual commerce, and the nature of the work itself, including the emotional labor involved. Some women who sell sex are exposed to regular physical and sexual violence in the course of their work; for other women who sell sex, violence is rare or nonexistent. Some women sell sex under the protection of law; other women sell sex under threat of arrest. Some women sell sex in the high-risk environment of crime-ridden streets; other women sell sex in luxury hotels. One thing that is true of most women who sell sex is that they encounter significant social stigma because of the work they do.

Given the differences in motivation and context, it is not surprising that differing levels of mental health concerns are seen among women who sell sex. In Chaps. 4 and 5, we reviewed the research on a variety of mental health concerns including post-traumatic stress disorder, anxiety, depression, suicide, and substance abuse. Our review found that, in most cases, samples of women who sell sex experience a higher prevalence of mental health concerns than women who do not sell sex. However, this does not mean that all women who sell sex have mental health problems. Nor do higher prevalence rates in themselves provide evidence that selling sex *causes* mental health concerns. Other factors contributing to the high prevalence may be that some women begin selling sex with pre-existing mental health disorders or with histories of physical, sexual, or substance abuse that increase their likelihood of developing psychological disorders.

In Chap. 6, we reviewed the literature on transitioning out of selling sex. Some women decide to stop selling sex after a violent encounter with a customer, to become sober, or through contact with the criminal justice system or an exit organization. Other women transition out of selling sex after completing higher education, saving enough money to start a business, or reaching an age where selling sex is not as profitable as it once was. Women stop selling sex for a variety of reasons, which we conceptualized in Chap. 6 as fitting into push and pull factors. Often multiple factors together influence a woman's decision to stop selling sex.

Is Selling Sex Psychologically Harmful to Women?

To be clear, this book has not focused on selling sex under coercion or in the context of human trafficking. We strongly believe that selling sex under these circumstances is a violation of basic human rights and is clearly harmful to women on many levels, including psychologically.

In Chap. 1, we acknowledged the controversy surrounding the question of whether or how commonly women can sell sex under free will circumstances. Although it is not possible to know the circumstances of every research participant, our goal was to review research of women who exerted some level of deliberate choice to sell sex. Our review of the literature among this population reveals a general trend whereby women selling sex have a higher prevalence of mental health concerns and drug use than women in the general population. Due to the inability to conduct experimental research, confounding factors, and a lack of prospective and longitudinal research designs and appropriate control samples, it is not possible to establish whether selling sex either directly or indirectly *causes* mental health problems. Based on the research conducted, it seems likely that the relationships are multi-directional, with selling sex contributing to mental health concerns for some women, mental health concerns contributing to the decision to sell sex for some women, and outside factors, such as trauma history or a lack of social support, contributing to some women both having mental health concerns and selling sex. Further, differentiating between these scenarios is not always simple. For example, even in situations where mental health symptoms seem to develop after the initiation of selling sex, it may be unclear whether subclinical levels of the mental health concerns existed prior, contributing to the development of the clinical levels of mental illness and possibly also contributing to the decision to sell sex. Text Box 8.1 provides a brief example of a complex case in which mental health factors and life circumstances interact in multiple ways with selling sex. This case example illustrates how many of the psychological factors reviewed in this book rarely present in isolation.

Text Box 8.1 Case Example Illustrating Complex Links Between Factors Influencing the Sale of Sex

Imagine a young woman who experiences a major depressive episode after the loss of a loved one. She begins self-medicating with illicit substances, which spirals into substance abuse. Her addiction elicits financial strain, which creates more stress. As her substance abuse progresses, she begins to sell sex to purchase drugs. Selling sex causes her to use more substances to escape from the stress of the double life she is now leading. Her addiction exacerbates her depression and results in a substance-induced anxiety disorder. In this scenario, depression is *both* a precursor and a consequence of selling sex and both depression and selling sex elicit a host of other mental health concerns.

A relevant factor in considering the links between selling sex and mental health concerns is that certain segments of women may bear a disproportionate amount of the psychological burdens of selling sex. The research is relatively clear that women with less education are more likely to sell sex than those with more education, and among women who sell sex, those with less education experience more mental health concerns (Burnette et al., 2008; El-Bassel, Simoni, Cooper, Gilbert, & Schilling, 2001; Hong, Li, Fang, & Zhao, 2007; Kramer & Berg, 2003; Marchand et al., 2012). Similarly, racial and ethnic minority women are more likely to sell sex than their counterparts, and tend to start selling sex at younger ages, which can also be a risk factor (Kramer & Berg, 2003; McClanahan, McClelland, Abram, & Teplin, 1999; Medrano et al., 2003). Further, socio-demographic factors are also associated with working in different types of settings; thus, this is another way that disparities in the mental health associations of selling sex can be compounded. Our review reveals a general trend whereby women selling sex outdoors have a higher prevalence of drug use and mental health concerns compared to women selling sex indoors. Street-level work, or selling sex outdoors, typically refers to where a commercial sex transaction originates rather than where it is consummated. The research literature is in agreement that selling sex outdoors subjects women to a heightened risk of physical and sexual violence, disease, and arrest, all of which can negatively impact psychological wellbeing. A small number of cities have implemented comprehensive harm reduction strategies to minimize the risks of selling sex outdoors, however, such efforts are exceedingly rare. We should note that, despite the risks of working outdoors, some qualitative research has shown that some women prefer street-level work over brothel or parlor work because it can offer greater autonomy as well as potential for increased earnings (e.g., Abel & Fitzgerald, 2012).

There is less agreement in the literature about whether selling sex in indoor settings is universally harmful. It is important to understand, as highlighted in Chap. 3, that even one category of venue, such as brothels, can pose substantial variations in structure, safety, compensation, and stressors. Our review indicates that *some* indoor environments appear to significantly reduce, though not entirely eliminate, the risks of selling sex present in outdoor environments. However, even the safest contexts pose some risks associated with multiple sexual partners, unknown customers, and, the attitudes and behaviors of venue managers or other stakeholders. Further, although the research has highlighted some differences in mental health outcomes based on the context in which sex is sold, it is important to realize that the boundaries between the various worksites are somewhat fluid, as women can move from one context to another, or simultaneously work in multiple settings. Finally, even though levels and types of stigma may differ based on the context in which sex is sold, nearly all women who sell sex experience substantial social stigma. As we discussed in Chap. 3, the negative effects of stigma can include isolation, personal relationship problems, and stress that can become psychologically harmful. Our review highlights the important role that social support plays in the mental health of women who sell sex. Social support seems to buffer against some of the emotional and psychological risks factors associated with selling sex.

Our review is clear that not all women who sell sex experience mental health concerns, but that some contexts, factors, and experiences associated with selling sex can increase mental health symptoms. This highlights the importance of having competent mental health care available to women who sell sex. We addressed this topic in Chap. 7.

Limitations of Our Approach and the Literature Reviewed

Overall, the risks to women who sell sex are often understood better from a physical health than mental health standpoint. More work remains to be done in understanding if and how the activity of selling sex impacts women psychologically and emotionally. This section summarizes some of the ways in which the existing literature is ill-equipped to address this topic. In addition, we highlight the methodological limitations inherent to our review.

Representativeness

As an introduction to the psychology of selling sex, this book is by no means exhaustive. When summarizing the empirical research, we sought to provide a balanced review that illustrates the great diversity of samples, settings, and findings present in the literature. However, this approach is not meant to imply that any of the particular samples or settings described is equally common either in the literature or in practice. The topics examined in the literature depend on the motivations, interests, and biases of the researchers as well as their access to samples. That is to say, the breadth of psychological research conducted does not represent the breadth of sexual commerce that takes place and cannot be assumed to be an overview of all forms of selling sex, nor a balanced sampling of populations.

To illustrate, much of the research on selling sex in the United States has been conducted using samples of women selling sex on the street, but this may not reflect the typical setting where sex is sold. Weitzer (2005a, b, 2009) has maintained that selling sex on the streets makes up roughly one-fifth of all prostitution in America and that selling sex indoors, although much more common, is less visible. This means that we may least understand the forms of selling sex that are the most common.

A similar concern regarding the representativeness of the research exists within the literature on indoor contexts. Much of the research on selling sex indoors has been conducted in high-income countries where indoor work is characterized by significantly reduced risk and relatively favorable conditions compared to selling sex on the street. However, sex is sold indoors throughout the world, not just in high-income locales. Although safer than street work, indoor venues in the developing world often operate under less favorable conditions than those in the United States or Europe (e.g., Jenkins & Rahman, 2002; Weitzer, 2009). Even within a given city or neighborhood, there can be significant differences in working conditions between indoor venues. Despite the application to many policy discussions, a simple dichotomous distinction between indoor and outdoor work does not necessarily reflect the many nuances and complexities of sexual commerce. More research on the variety of indoor environments is greatly needed.

Samples and Scope

Throughout this book, we have focused exclusively on cisgender women. The experiences of men and transgendered individuals who sell sex may differ in many regards from the literature reviewed in this book. There is a growing body of research giving voice to men and transgendered individuals who sell sex (e.g., Baral et al., 2015; Minichiello et al., 2002; Ocha & Earth, 2013); still, rigorous psychological research on these populations is lacking. Further, in his 2009 review, Weitzer noted that almost all research on sex work is gender-specific, with very few studies comparing the experiences of women and men who sell at the same level or in similar work environments. Given this, comparative gender studies focusing on the psychological aspects of selling sex would be particularly informative.

Our review has also focused exclusively on adult women who sell sex voluntarily. We did not explore human trafficking or the commercial sexual exploitation of children. Both are extremely critical issues that have attracted much research interest. Ongoing work in these areas is essential.

We also did not review the psychological motivations, experiences, and outcomes of those who purchase sex. Although there has been some research on customers, especially male customers, most of it has been conducted using a sociological or criminological lens rather than a psychological one. The psychology of *buying* sex is an important topic for future research and will contribute to a deeper understanding of commercial sex.

Quality of Research Reviewed

As noted in Chap. 1, well-designed research that compares the psychological experiences and outcomes of women selling sex to women in appropriate control groups is very rare, but we have attempted to highlight such studies throughout this review whenever possible. We have also incorporated findings from peer-reviewed studies with simpler designs in our review, noting key limitations when relevant. Some of these methodological limitations are due to the difficulties inherent in gathering empirical data on women selling sex. These include the stigmatized nature of the work and the fact that women who sell sex are often a hidden population. Not only is it difficult to identify potential research participants, it can also be difficult to convince them to participate in research.

Additionally, there is an ongoing debate in the field about how researchers' ideological biases inform the quality of research. For example, in an exchange in a special forum in the journal, *Violence Against Women* (2005a, b), Weitzer criticized anti-prostitution researchers for selectively citing the literature to advance their agendas, failing to adequately describe their samples and how participants were recruited, failing to use appropriate control groups, and failing to fully disclose their research procedures and questionnaires. He argued that: "*In no area* of the social sciences has ideology contaminated knowledge more pervasively than in writings on the sex industry. Too often in this area, the canons of scientific inquiry are suspended and research deliberately skewed to serve a particular political agenda" (2005a, p. 934). Farley (2005) and Raphael and Shapiro (2005), who were among those criticized by Weitzer, responded in part by challenging some of Weitzer's claims and in part by highlighting the challenges of conducting research among women who sell sex, which we have already reviewed. This exchange is emblematic of the deep disagreements that exist in this field of research and it highlights how researchers' biases can be particularly salient, given the potentially impactful political, social, and moral conclusions that may be drawn from the work, as well as the associated values that may be driving the research. On the basis of our review, we can highlight that the poor quality research we encountered was not limited to research from a single ideology. Regardless of the political lens, we encountered studies that failed to meet the basic scientific reporting standards common in mainstream psychological research. For example, in some studies it was unclear how mental health variables were assessed. Other studies failed to adequately describe the samples (e.g., age, work environment, etc.). Use of appropriate control groups was the exception rather than the rule across the board.

Future Methodological Directions

Almost all research examining psychological topics among women selling sex has been cross-sectional in nature. Most longitudinal data on women selling sex are epidemiological rather than psychological in nature. Potterat, Rothenberg, Muth, Darrow, and Phillips-Plummer (1998) and Potterat et al. 2004) deserve immense credit for their extensive undertakings in this area. Now there is a great need for research that measures the psychological experiences and mental health outcomes of women selling sex over extended periods of time. These types of data are extremely challenging to collect under the best of circumstances. Such data collection procedures are daunting due to the financial and research resources required, the challenges of long-term follow up in a stigmatized and often transient population, and associated participant attrition. However, if conducted, this type of research would offer enormous benefits for scholars, clinicians, policymakers, and women who sell sex in answering important questions, such as: Is the psychological experience of selling sex stable or variable? Do mental health concerns increase, decrease, or remain stable over the course of selling sex or after transitioning out of selling sex? How do key life events impact the psychological experience of selling sex? What therapeutic interventions are effective in the long-term among women who sell sex? Current research is ill-equipped to answer these questions.

In addition to long-term research, there would be a benefit to more systematic reviews. Within psychology, management, and medicine, systematic reviews and meta-analyses have helped synthesize seemingly conflicting research results. Although integrative reviews, systematic reviews, and meta-analyses have examined selling sex in relation to alcohol use (Li, Li, & Stanton, 2010), HIV prevalence (Baral et al., 2012), and sex work laws and health outcomes (Platt et al., 2018), systematic reviews and meta-analyses examining the relationship between selling sex and key mental health concerns are noticeably lacking. This presents a significant opportunity for future research.

Topical Suggestions for Future Research on Women Who Sell Sex

Sexually Transmitted Infections and Mental Health

Because of our specific emphasis on psychology, we excluded from our review the vast epidemiology and public health literatures on the prevalence of HIV and other sexually transmitted infections (STIs) among women who sell sex. However, there are clear areas of intersection between STIs and mental health. For example, research has shown that individuals with a serious mental illness have an increased risk of acquiring sexually transmitted diseases (Carey, Carey, & Kalichman, 1997).

This is a topic to be explored in future research among women selling sex, given the increased prevalence of certain mental health conditions among women who sell sex. In addition, sexually transmitted diseases could impact the psychological motivations, experiences, and outcomes of women who sell sex. For example, fear of contracting a sexually transmitted disease could lead to higher levels of anxiety, and being diagnosed with HIV could lead to depression. Indeed, meta-analytic research within the general population has found that HIV infection is linked to increased risk for major depressive disorder (Ciesla & Roberts, 2001).

The literature reviewed in Chap. 4 showed that women selling sex had a higher prevalence of depression than women in the general population (and a similar prevalence of depression to women substance users who had not sold sex). In this book, we have considered primarily psychological, social, and structural causes of depression among women who sell sex. However, a point for consideration is that a growing body of evidence suggests that some cases of depression have biological origins. Specifically, when faced with a viral, bacterial, or parasitic infection, the body coordinates an immune response that involves the production of proinflammatory cytokines whose presence is linked to depressive symptoms (Dantzer et al., 2008; Miller, Maletic, & Raison, 2009). Meta-analysis has shown that these cytokines, specifically TNF-α and IL-6, are present in higher concentrations in individuals with depression compared to individuals in control populations (Dowlati et al., 2010). Given that selling sex involves intimate contact with customers, it raises the likelihood of infection, even when protection is used. It is possible that some cases of depression or other mental health concerns among women selling sex might be related, in part, to the presence of infections, sexually transmitted or otherwise. Empirical research is needed to determine if, and to what extent, this is the case. This possibility underscores the need for coordinated care and research between psychological, medical, and public health practitioners.

Night Work and Depression

Sexual commerce is a key component of the night-time economy, and many women selling sex work primarily or exclusively during the evening or late-night hours (although some women also experience steady demand in the early morning hours before customers go to work, e.g., Dalla, 2002). Recent research reviews have found that working at night is linked with an increased likelihood of depression (Angerer, Schmook, Elfantel, & Li, 2017; Lee et al., 2017). One possible mechanism for this relationship is that individuals working at night are exposed to less sunlight than those working during the day. Reduced exposure to sunlight can lead to vitamin D deficiency (Holick, 2007), which in turn has been linked to higher risk for depression (Anglin, Samaan, Walter, & McDonald, 2013; Berk et al., 2007). Thus, it is possible that the increased prevalence of depression among women selling sex might be attributable, in part, to the particular hours that women work. Although this possibility has not yet been empirically examined, this line of inquiry may yield insight into a potential causal mechanism for the relationship between selling sex and depression.

Harm Reduction

Many in the mental health, social work, medical, and public health communities have advocated for a harm reduction approach when addressing difficult social problems such as substance abuse and HIV (e.g., MacCoun, 1998; Marlatt, 1996; Marlatt, Larimer, & Witkiewitz, 2012). Harm reduction seeks to modify behaviors in order to minimize risk. For example, drug abuse harm reduction strategies have included needle exchange programs to reduce the spread of infection and disease from shared needles and naloxone programs to reduce the risk of overdose. As we have noted throughout this book, selling sex can involve considerable risk (e.g., violence, drug use, disease). These risks are higher when sex is sold on the street; yet, indoor work environments are not risk-free (e.g., Weitzer, 2009). Given this, a number of harm reduction strategies have been developed to minimize risks for women who sell sex. These strategies include sex education, condom-negotiation skills training, safety training, customer registries, and empowerment initiatives (see Rekart, 2005 for a review).

Psychologists and other mental health practitioners have made significant contributions to harm reduction efforts in the areas of drug abuse and disease prevention, some of which specifically target women who sell sex. However, there remains an opportunity to develop harm reduction interventions that target specific mental health concerns for women who sell sex. That is, in settings where the risk for mental health concerns is high among women selling sex, prevention programs could be developed and implemented to proactively reduce the likelihood of concerns developing as opposed to reactively addressing concerns only after they emerge or become severe enough to require treatment. Such prophylactic mental health interventions would require a significant investment of resources, but could also produce significant benefits. Any such interventions should be based on empirical evidence and be subjected to rigorous evaluation, all the while keeping the welfare of women who sell sex at the forefront.

Industrial-Organizational (I-O) Psychology and Related Disciplines

Almost none of the research on women who sell sex has been conducted within the field of I-O psychology or related disciplines such as organizational behavior or human resources management. This is perhaps the result of the controversy surrounding the characterization of selling sex as work. Those who argue that selling sex should be legal or decriminalized sometimes maintain that selling sex should be considered a job like any other job. Those who argue for the abolition of commercial sex typically reach the opposite conclusion—selling sex is not like other forms of employment and perhaps should not be considered work at all.

Selling sex, when voluntary and not coerced, has some things in common with many forms of work, including that it involves the exchange of money for a service and that women must advertise their services, secure and/or travel to a work location, and negotiate with customers. Similar to service professions, selling sex involves close physical contact and requires significant emotional labor. For these reasons, selling sex could be considered a job, though in some circumstances it is an undesirable or even harmful job, as is true of certain other occupations.

On the other hand, it is difficult to argue that selling sex is a job *like any other job*. This is not an argument against providing those who sell sex with the rights and protections of other humans and workers. It is simply an acknowledgment that, in our estimation, the unique characteristics of selling sex outweigh the commonalities with other occupations, suggesting that it may be considered a job, but is not a job *like any other*. First, although it has some things in common with traditional service occupations, it involves a physical intimacy that is not seen in other forms of work. Second, it is illegal in many locations, which immediately differentiates it from the majority of other occupations that are legal. Third, few occupations, even ones involving quasi-legal or illegal activities, encounter the degree of stigma that selling sex does. Even where selling sex is legal, it is still stigmatized, though to a lesser degree than where it is prohibited by law. For all of these reasons, selling sex often involves a level of risk not present in the great majority of occupations.

Bruckert and Parent's (2018) edited volume on third-party management in the sex industry is a recent exception to the absence of selling sex as a topic within the disciplines of I-O psychology or management. However, its contributors are primarily from the area of criminology rather than psychology and management. I-O psychologists and management scholars have not been afraid to investigate atypical occupations. For example, research in *Administrative Science Quarterly*, a top-tier management journal, has examined bill collectors (Sutton, 1991), symphony musicians (Allmendinger & Hackman, 1996), zookeepers (Bunderson & Thompson, 2009), circus professionals (Berg, 2016), and nuns in a Roman Catholic order (Bartunek, 1984). However, women who sell sex are notably missing even though their numbers likely exceed those in each of the aforementioned occupations. The disciplines of I-O psychology, organizational behavior, and human resource management seek to understand work from the perspective of both workers and organizations. This approach complements the medical and clinical approaches that currently dominate the research landscape. Perhaps scholars in these disciples are deterred by the stigma associated with studying the sex industry, or by the difficulty in collecting data from hidden populations. I-O psychology and management frameworks and tools may provide an opportunity for future research that could make a meaningful contribution to our understanding of the psychology of selling sex.

Mind-Body-Spirit Theories

In addition to the discipline of I-O psychology just noted, the discipline of psychology of religion could make a unique contributing to understanding the psychology of selling sex. Not much is known about the religious or spiritual orientations of women who sell sex, but there is no reason to believe that religion and/or spirituality are not important to women who sell sex. Spiritual struggles may be a relevant theme for exploration. A number of distinct forms of spiritual struggles have been delineated (Pargament, 2007). To the extent that selling sex may conflict with religious or spiritual beliefs, values, and morals, women may experience some of these spiritual struggles, such as fear and concern about divine punishment, feeling rejected by God, concern about moral imperfections, interpersonal conflict about selling sex on religious grounds, or feeling rejected or offended by religious individuals. Research is needed to establish if, and to what extent, spiritual struggles are present among women who sell sex. Research has supported links between spiritual struggles and mental health symptoms, including anxiety, depression, anger, negative mood, guilt, and social dysfunction (see Exline, 2013). Thus, spiritual struggles among some women who sell sex may help to account for some of the great variability in mental health outcomes observed in the literature among women who sell sex.

Religion and spirituality will not be relevant to all women who sell sex. Beyond the theoretical framework of religion and spirituality, additional work can be done to examine commercial sex through the lens of other cultural and philosophical theories of the human body and sexuality. As noted, the mental health outcomes of selling sex tend to differ from one woman to the next. This may, in part, be due to cultural and philosophical differences in the way women think about their bodies, sexuality, and commercial sex. Along these lines, some research questions ripe for investigation include: Do women who ascribe to a mind-body-spirit connection experience selling sex differently than their counterparts? How do various moral conceptualizations of selling sex impact psychological wellbeing among women who sell sex? And, how do a woman's cultural perspectives of commercial sex impact levels of acceptance versus dissonance experienced about the choice to sell sex?

Discussion

Much of the scholarly discussion on selling sex has been polemic and divisive. This is both understandable, given the high stakes involved, and unfortunate, because it can hinder advances in scientific knowledge. As a discipline, psychology aspires to provide benefit to others, ensure accuracy and truthfulness in science, promote justice, and respect people's rights and dignity (American Psychological Association, 2017). We have sought to adhere to these principles in our review. In this volume, we have reviewed the research literature on the psychology of selling sex, specifically focusing on women. The goal of this book has been to provide a broad picture of the current psychological knowledge base, rather than to review or advocate for research fitting only a particular ideology about selling sex. In adopting this approach, we acknowledge that those with strong ideologies about selling sex may criticize our decision to include research conducted by those with different ideologies from their own.

As discussed throughout this book, our review suggests that selling sex is a complex, multi-faceted phenomenon. This makes it problematic to extrapolate findings from one setting to another or to broadly generalize about the psychological motivations, experiences, and outcomes of women who sell sex.

In this chapter, we have presented the limitations of our review as well as the limitations of the body of literature, which highlight a need for research findings to be interpreted with caution. We also identified areas where there is both opportunity and need for additional research. Some of these ideas are purposefully speculative and are intended to illustrate how research on the psychology of selling sex can be linked with existing work in other disciplines. We encourage students, researchers, mental health practitioners, and policymakers to draw on psychology to further the existing understanding of sexual commerce and to ultimately improve the welfare of women for whom this is a relevant topic.

References

Abel, G. M., & Fitzgerald, L. J. (2012). 'The street's got its advantages': Movement between sectors of the sex industry in a decriminalised environment. *Health, Risk & Society, 14,* 7–23. https://doi.org/10.1080/13698575.2011.640664.

Allmendinger, J., & Hackman, J. R. (1996). Organizations in changing environments: The case of East German symphony orchestras. *Administrative Science Quarterly, 41,* 337–369. https://doi.org/10.2307/2393935.

American Psychological Association. (2017). *Ethical principles of psychologists and code of conduct.* Washington, DC: Author. Retrieved from https://www.apa.org/ethics/code/ethics-code-2017.pdf.

Angerer, P., Schmook, R., Elfantel, I., & Li, J. (2017). Night work and the risk of depression: A systematic review. *Deutsches Aerzteblatt International, 114,* 404–411. https://doi.org/10.3238/arztebl.2017.0404.

Anglin, R. E. S., Samaan, Z., Walter, S. D., & McDonald, S. D. (2013). Vitamin D deficiency and depression in adults: systematic review and meta-analysis. *British Journal of Psychiatry, 202,* 100–107. https://doi.org/10.1192/bjp.bp.111.106666.

Baral, S., Beyrer, C., Muessig, K., Poteat, T., Wirtz, A. L., Decker, M. R., … Kerrigan, D. (2012). Burden of HIV among female sex workers in low-income and middle-income countries: a systematic review and meta-analysis. *Lancet Infectious Diseases, 12,* 538–549. https://doi.org/10.1016/s1473-3099(12)70066-x.

Baral, S. D., Friedman, M. R., Geibel, S., Rebe, K., Bozhinov, B., Diouf, D., … Cáceres, C. F. (2015). Male sex workers: Practices, contexts, and vulnerabilities for HIV acquisition and transmission. *Lancet, 385,* 260–273. https://doi.org/10.1016/s0140-6736(14)60801-1.

Bartunek, J. M. (1984). Changing interpretive schemes and organizational restructuring: The example of a religious order. *Administrative Science Quarterly, 29,* 355–372. https://doi.org/10.2307/2393029.

Berg, J. M. (2016). Balancing on the creative highwire. *Administrative Science Quarterly, 61,* 433–468. https://doi.org/10.1177/0001839216642211.

Berk, M., Sanders, K. M., Pasco, J. A., Jacka, F. N., Williams, L. J., Hayles, A. L., et al. (2007). Vitamin D deficiency may play a role in depression. *Medical Hypotheses, 69,* 1316–1319. https://doi.org/10.1016/j.mehy.2007.04.001.

Bruckert, C., & Parent, C. (Eds.). (2018). *Getting past 'the Pimp': Management in the sex industry.* Toronto: University of Toronto Press.

Bunderson, J. S., & Thompson, J. A. (2009). The call of the wild: Zookeepers, callings, and the double-edged sword of deeply meaningful work. *Administrative Science Quarterly, 54,* 32–57. https://doi.org/10.2189/asqu.2009.54.1.32.

Burnette, M. L., Lucas, E., Ilgen, M., Frayne, S. M., Mayo, J., & Weitlauf, J. C. (2008). Prevalence and health correlates of prostitution among patients entering treatment for substance use disorders. *Archives of General Psychiatry, 65,* 337–344. https://doi.org/10.1001/archpsyc.65.3.337.

Carey, M. P., Carey, K. B., & Kalichman, S. C. (1997). Risk for human immunodeficiency virus (HIV) infection among persons with severe mental illnesses. *Clinical Psychology Review, 17,* 271–291. https://doi.org/10.1016/s0272-7358(97)00019-6.

Ciesla, J. A., & Roberts, J. E. (2001). Meta-analysis of the relationship between HIV infection and risk for depressive disorders. *American Journal of Psychiatry, 158,* 725–730. https://doi.org/10.1176/appi.ajp.158.5.725.

Dalla, R. L. (2002). Night moves: A qualitative investigation of street-level sex work. *Psychology of Women Quarterly, 26,* 63–73. https://doi.org/10.1111/1471-6402.00044.

Dantzer, R., O'Connor, J. C., Freund, G. G., Johnson, R. W., & Kelley, K. W. (2008). From inflammation to sickness and depression: When the immune system subjugates the brain. *Nature Reviews Neuroscience, 9,* 46–56. https://doi.org/10.1038/nrn2297.

Dowlati, Y., Herrmann, N., Swardfager, W., Liu, H., Sham, L., Reim, E. K., et al. (2010). A meta-analysis of cytokines in major depression. *Biological Psychiatry, 67,* 446–457. https://doi.org/10.1016/j.biopsych.2009.09.033.

El-Bassel, N., Simoni, J. M., Cooper, D. K., Gilbert, L., & Schilling, R. F. (2001). Sex trading and psychological distress among women on methadone. *Psychology of Addictive Behaviors, 15,* 177–184. https://doi.org/10.1037//0893-164X.15.3.177.

Exline, J. J. (2013). Religious and spiritual struggles. In J. J. Exline, K. I. Pargament, & J. W. Jones (Eds.), *APA handbook of psychology, religion, and spirituality (Vol 1): Context, theory, and research* (pp. 459–475). American Psychological Association. https://doi.org/10.1037/14045-025.

Farley, M. (2005). Prostitution harms women even if indoors: Reply to Weitzer. *Violence Against Women, 11,* 950–964. https://doi.org/10.1177/1077801205276987.

Holick, M. F. (2007). Vitamin D deficiency. *New England Journal of Medicine, 357*(3), 266–281. https://doi.org/10.1056/nejmra070553.

Hong, Y., Li, X., Fang, X., & Zhao, R. (2007). Correlates of suicidal ideation and attempt among female sex workers in China. *Health Care for Women International, 28,* 490–505. https://doi.org/10.1080/07399330701226529.

Jenkins, C., & Rahman, H. (2002). Rapidly Changing Conditions in the Brothels of Bangladesh: Impact on HIV/STD. *AIDS Education and Prevention, 14*(3_supplement), 97–106. https://doi.org/10.1521/aeap.14.4.97.23882

Kramer, L. A., & Berg, E. C. (2003). A survival analysis of timing of entry into prostitution: The differential impact of race, educational level, and childhood/adolescent risk factors. *Sociological Inquiry, 73,* 511–528. https://doi.org/10.1111/1475-682X.00069.

Lee, A., Myung, S.-K., Cho, J. J., Jung, Y.-J., Yoon, J. L., & Kim, M. Y. (2017). Night shift work and risk of depression: Meta-analysis of observational studies. *Journal of Korean Medical Science, 32,* 1091–1096. https://doi.org/10.3346/jkms.2017.32.7.1091.

Li, Q., Li, X., & Stanton, B. (2010). Alcohol use among female sex workers and male clients: An integrative review of global literature. *Alcohol and Alcoholism, 45,* 188–199. https://doi.org/10.1093/alcalc/agp095.

MacCoun, R. J. (1998). Toward a psychology of harm reduction. *American Psychologist, 53,* 1199–1208. https://doi.org/10.1037/0003-066x.53.11.1199.

Marchand, K., Oviedo-Joekes, E., Guh, D., Marsh, D. C., Brissette, S., & Schechter, M. T. (2012). Sex work involvement among women with long-term opioid injection drug dependence who enter opioid agonist treatment. *Harm Reduction Journal, 9*. https://doi.org/10.1186/1477-7517-9-8.

Marlatt, G. A. (1996). Harm reduction: Come as you are. *Addictive Behaviors, 21,* 779–788. https://doi.org/10.1016/0306-4603(96)00042-1.

Marlatt, G. A., Larimer, M. E., & Witkiewitz, K. E. (Eds.). (2012). *Harm reduction: Pragmatic strategies for managing high-risk behaviors* (2nd ed.). New York: Guilford.

McClanahan, S. F., McClelland, G. M., Abram, K. M., & Teplin, L. A. (1999). Pathways into prostitution among female jail detainees and their implications for mental health service. *Psychiatric Services, 50,* 1606–1613. https://doi.org/10.1176/ps.50.12.1606.

Medrano, M. A., Hatch, J. P., Zule, W. A., & Desmond, D. P. (2003). Childhood trauma and adult prostitution behavior in a multiethnic heterosexual drug-using population. *American Journal of Drug & Alcohol Abuse, 29*(2), 463–486. https://doi.org/10.1081/ada-120020527

Miller, A. H., Maletic, V., & Raison, C. L. (2009). Inflammation and its discontents: The role of cytokines in the pathophysiology of major depression. *Biological Psychiatry, 65,* 732–741. https://doi.org/10.1016/j.biopsych.2008.11.029.

Minichiello, V., Marino, R., Browne, J., Jamieson, M., Peterson, K., Reuter, B., et al. (2002). Male sex workers in three Australian cities. *Journal of Homosexuality, 42,* 29–51. https://doi.org/10.1300/j082v42n01_02.

Ocha, W., & Earth, B. (2013). Identity diversification among transgender sex workers in Thailand's sex tourism industry. *Sexualities, 16,* 195–216. https://doi.org/10.1177/1363460712471117.

Pargament, K. I. (2007). *Spiritually integrated psychotherapy: Understanding and addressing the sacred*. New York, NY: Guilford Press.

Platt, L., Grenfell, P., Meiksin, R., Elmes, J., Sherman, S. G., Sanders, T., … Crago, A.-L. (2018). Associations between sex work laws and sex workers' health: A systematic review and meta-analysis of quantitative and qualitative studies. *PLOS Medicine, 15*(12), e1002680. https://doi.org/10.1371/journal.pmed.1002680.

Potterat, J. J., Rothenberg, R. B., Muth, S. Q., Darrow, W. W., & Phillips-Plummer, L. (1998). Pathways to prostitution: The chronology of sexual and drug abuse milestones. *Journal of Sex Research, 35,* 333–340. https://doi.org/10.1080/00224499809551951.

Potterat, J. J., Brewer, D., Muth, S. Q., Rothenberg, R. B., Woodhouse, D. E., Muth, J. B., et al. (2004). Mortality in a long-term open cohort of prostitute women. *American Journal of Epidemiology, 159,* 778–785. https://doi.org/10.1093/aje/kwh110.

Raphael, J., & Shapiro, D. L. (2005). Reply to Weitzer. *Violence Against Women, 11,* 965–970. https://doi.org/10.1177/1077801205277041.

Rekart, M. L. (2005). Sex-work harm reduction. *Lancet, 366,* 2123–2134. https://doi.org/10.1016/s0140-6736(05)67732-x.

Sutton, R. I. (1991). Maintaining norms about expressed emotions: The case of bill collectors. *Administrative Science Quarterly, 36,* 245. https://doi.org/10.2307/2393355.

Weitzer, R. (2005a). Flawed theory and method in studies of prostitution. *Violence Against Women, 11,* 934–949. https://doi.org/10.1177/1077801205276986.

Weitzer, R. (2005b). Rehashing tired claims about prostitution: A Response to Farley and Raphael and Shapiro. *Violence Against Women, 11,* 971–977. https://doi.org/10.1177/1077801205277090.

Weitzer, R. (2009). Sociology of sex work. *Annual Review of Sociology, 35,* 213–234. https://doi.org/10.1146/annurev-soc-070308-120025.

Weitzer, R. (2010). *Sex for sale: Prostitution, pornography, and the sex industry* (2nd ed.). New York: Routledge.

Widom, C., & Kuhns, J. B. (1996). Childhood victimization and subsequent risk for promiscuity, prostitution, and teenage pregnancy: A prospective study. *American Journal of Public Health, 86,* 1607–1612. https://doi.org/10.2105/ajph.86.11.1607.

The manufacturer's authorised representative in the EU is Springer Nature Customer Service Centre GmbH, Europaplatz 3, 69115 Heidelberg, Germany. If you have any concerns regarding our products, please contact ProductSafety@springernature.com

Printed and bound by CPI Group (UK) Ltd, Croydon, CR0 4YY
30/09/2026
02225696-0008